Praise for *Running with a*

"A stylish and sparkly writer."—*The New York Times*

"Every new runner worries that she will finish last in her first race. Jill Grunenwald has actually done it and is here to report that last place isn't nearly as bad as it seems (unless they've already boxed up the bananas). Read Jill's fun and feisty memoir for the inspiration, for the laughs, and for the truth about what it's like at the back of the pack. She may not be fast (yet), but she's a blast, and she'll motivate you to run, too." —Jennifer Graham, author of *Honey, Do You Need a Ride? Confessions of a Fat Runner*

"What does a serious runner look like? Someone who follows a training plan, runs regardless of weather, travels to races, keeps track of her times, and would never call herself a jogger. Jill Grunenwald looks— and runs—like a serious runner." —Rachel Toor, author of *Personal Record: A Love Affair with Running*

"*Running with a Police Escort* is a manifesto for every out-of-shape middle school girl who came in last running the mile and decided from that point forward that she was just not meant to be a runner. In this hilarious and relatable tale of the journey from couch potato to half marathon, Jill Grunenwald will inspire you to lace up your running shoes, step out of your comfort zone and laugh your way all the way to the finish line." —Jill Angie, author of *Running With Curves* and *Not Your Average Half Marathon*

"*Running with a Police Escort* is for anyone who has ever struggled with any challenge, physical or mental. Her stories of racing at the back of the pack are relatable to any runner, but even if you've never considered running at all, you'll want to read this book. Jill's love of Cleveland and her hilarious asides will keep you turning the pages to find out what happens in the next race." —Stephani Itibrout, PBS Digital Innovator and Cleveland Rite Aid Marathon Ambassador

"Jill Grunenwald is fantastic at conveying the heart of an authentic runner. She humorously voices the lessons, fears, joys, race-day blunders, and head games every runner can appreciate. *Running with a Police Escort* is a relatable reminder of how the passion and influence of the run can take root and shape life, allowing one to reach beyond their wildest expectations." —Jackie Dikos, columnist for *Runner's World* and author *Finish Line Fueling*

"No matter the challenge, readers witness her walking and finishing last with dignity. Readers can count on Grunenwald to be honest about herself and others, and sprinkled in the chapters are fun references to writers such as Joyce Carol Oates and Stephen King (she is a librarian, after all). This autobiography will appeal to and inspire those struggling to get healthy." —*Publisher's Weekly*

"Whether she's writing about setting goals, finding the best sports bra ("Strap. That. Shit. Down"), or getting out of a running slump, self-proclaimed slow runner Grunenwald's chatty, confessional style will entertain readers and perhaps even inspire them to lace up, too... Readers will find that the author's unique perspective "from the back of the pack" challenges preconceived notions as it encourages stepping outside of one's comfort zones." —*Booklist*

"[Jill] also is upbeat and funny. She's positive and sassy, a fun voice to read with an inspiring story to tell." —*Women's Running* magazine

"For everyone who's ever said they're too heavy to run, Jill's memoir is here to prove you wrong." —*Family Circle*

"Candid and laugh-out-loud [funny]." —Library Moments blog

Running

with a Police

Escort

Running
with a Police
Tales from the Back of the Pack
Escort

JILL GRUNENWALD

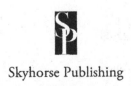

Skyhorse Publishing

Copyright © 2017, 2019 by Jill A. Grunenwald

All rights reserved. No part of this book may be reproduced in any manner without the express written consent of the publisher, except in the case of brief excerpts in critical reviews or articles. All inquiries should be addressed to Skyhorse Publishing, 307 West 36th Street, 11th Floor, New York, NY 10018.

Skyhorse Publishing books may be purchased in bulk at special discounts for sales promotion, corporate gifts, fund-raising, or educational purposes. Special editions can also be created to specifications. For details, contact the Special Sales Department, Skyhorse Publishing, 307 West 36th Street, 11th Floor, New York, NY 10018 or info@skyhorsepublishing.com.

Skyhorse® and Skyhorse Publishing® are registered trademarks of Skyhorse Publishing, Inc.®, a Delaware corporation.

Visit our website at www.skyhorsepublishing.com.

10 9 8 7 6 5 4 3 2 1

Library of Congress Cataloging-in-Publication Data is available on file.

Cover design by Tom Lau
Cover photo credit: Jill Grunenwald

Print ISBN: 978-1-5107-4091-4
Ebook ISBN: 978-1-5107-4092-1
Previous edition: 978-1-5107-1279-9

Printed in the United States of America

To Ben.
Life is a marathon and I'm so
happy I get to run it with you.

CONTENTS

AUTHOR'S NOTE

Memoirs are works of nonfiction and I have tried to make this story as true and honest as I can, often relying on blog posts I wrote at the time of events to assist in jogging my memory (pun intended). In some instances, timelines have been compressed and characters combined. Dialogue has been recreated to the best of my knowledge.

Every morning in Africa, a gazelle wakes up.
It knows it must run faster than the fastest lion or it will be killed.
Every morning in Africa, a lion wakes up.
It knows it must outrun the slowest gazelle or it will starve to death.
It doesn't matter whether you are a lion or a gazelle:
When the sun comes up, you'd better be running.

—African Proverb

I don't care for the damage that's been done,
but I don't mind the woman I've become.
Who is this woman I've become?

—Maura Rogers & The Bellows,
"This Woman"

INTRODUCTION

The decision to wear a one-piece Batman bodysuit to the race seemed like a brilliant idea until the moment I had to pee.

I've always had a strange affinity for Batman. Well, not so much Batman as Batgirl. As far as comic books and graphic novels go, my knowledge is limited and mostly gained through the osmosis of dating fellow self-identified geeks. But Batgirl, under her Barbara Gordon alias, worked as a librarian, like me.

I had entered the Running the Bridges Race with zero expectations. I'd really only registered because it was being hosted by Harness Cycle, the indoor cycling studio up the street from my apartment. Since they opened in the fall of 2013, I'd been a regular fixture in the early morning spin classes and had made a visit there a weekly part of my training when I ran my second half marathon back in the spring of 2014, a half marathon that ended with me walking the final third of the race because of a tweaked ankle.

That was May. It was now October and my relationship with running had been on a break the past six months. I'd wake up and see my neglected New Balance shoes eyeing me mournfully from the closet, and I'd assure them that I was just having trouble sleeping and this was just a case of insomnia, only to then sneak out and go to spinning or yoga instead of going for a run. After, I'd come home and they'd still be sitting in the exact same spot, tongues wagging in admonishment, and I'd promise them that I'd never, ever do it again; until, of course, I did it again.

Eventually like any amateur cheater, the guilt got to me, so when Harness Cycle announced they were hosting the 3.5-mile road race, Running the Bridges, I immediately signed up.

My hometown of Cleveland is a city of bridges, a veritable Venice of the Midwest. It is a city divided by the grand Cuyahoga River, which bends and breaks its way through the downtown district, creating fierce lines of loyalty depending on which side of the river you call home. The Running the Bridges course started at the studio and took runners over several of these bridges, from the fierce Veterans Memorial to the stoic Lorain-Carnegie, looping back to the studio, which is located in the Ohio City neighborhood.

It was at the start, standing in the stall of the on-site bathroom, that I realized the fatal flaw in my decision to dress in costume. It wasn't just that I had to unpin my bib to pee, it was that I had to unpin and then zip and strip in order to pee. I was basically wearing the adult version of footie pajamas—not a garment meant for a serious runner to wear to a race. I mean, there was a fucking cape attached, okay? And this was certainly not a garment designed to be worn by a runner as well-endowed as myself. The cheap zipper, which ended up completely breaking about a month later, kept creeping lower and lower as I ran, which meant I spent half the race tugging it back up, lest I flash the entire security team along the route.

With apologies to Billy Idol, and comparisons to Janet Jackson aside, it was a nice day for a wardrobe malfunction.

So there I was: running in a race I wasn't entirely sure I wanted to run, dressed as a caped crusader, in a costume that was constantly on the verge of unleashing my own personal superpowers with each bounced step.

At the course marker for Mile One, my friend Gina stood with a stopwatch, calling out numbers to let us runners know what our time was. She waved as I passed and I took the opportunity to sneak a peek over my shoulder. Call it silly and maybe even a little bit petty, but as a slower runner I always like to gauge where I am in relation to the rest of the pack. This race, however, the only thing back there was the police escort car as it slowly crawled behind me.

Oh, look. I was in last place.

Cleveland is a city that likes to sleep in. Especially on the weekends and especially in the fall and winter when the cold wind snaps at our windows, leaving us cozy and cocooned beneath the warm blankets on our beds.

This meant that for the next two and a half miles I had the entire city to myself, save for the police officers who stood along the sidewalks like centurions guiding me home.

If you ever want to feel like a superhero, I mean really feel like a superhero, figure out a way to shut down an entire city street and just run your little heart out with Gotham's finest standing guard. Bonus points if you dressed for the occasion, and it's a windy day, and you actually get some height on that cape.

It was during this moment of nirvana that I happened to see one of the policemen on the street gesture to get my attention and point to the car following me. I pulled out my earbuds and from the sidewalk he called out with a supportive smile, "You must be a very important person to have a police escort!"

With a grin, I popped my earbuds back in, gave him a thumbs-up, and continued on my way.

Around Mile Three, with only half a mile left until the finish line, I turned a corner and spotted Gina on a bicycle heading back towards the finish line, her volunteering done. Because this was my first real run in months, I found myself needing to walk more than usual, especially towards the end. When she saw me, Gina hopped off her bike and asked if she could walk with me.

Gina is a fellow runner, and she actually looks like one. She's petite, but has an athletic build and is a certified indoor cycling instructor. She literally works out for a living. On the other hand, I'm the voluptuous Batman. While walking at a quick clip we chatted about running and racing and life, the police car still slowly following us. Then, with maybe a quarter of a mile left, I looked up ahead and saw my boyfriend and dad waiting near the finish line. With a wave of goodbye, I picked up my pace and bolted towards that finish, channeling my inner superhero, cape flying high behind me.

I soon learned that out of the 169 entrants in the race, I was the last one to cross that line.

The thing about coming in last place is that all it really means is that of all the people who showed up that day, I just happened to be the slowest. That's it. Sure, I technically maybe may have "lost" the race, but that doesn't mean I'm a loser or anything. I still ran the same distance as the top finishers, it just took me a little bit longer to do it.

And here's the flip side of all of that: That race? The big event that everyone paid and showed up for? It couldn't end without me. Those faster runners who consistently win in their age group, were able to finish, grab their post-race fuel and medals, and go about their day. But those of us in the back, those of us who are on the slower side, who need a bit more time to cover the same amount of distance, we're the ones who bring that race home. Like that officer on the route said, we are very important people—at least in that context. When you think about it, we're pretty fucking cool.

Which is why being the final runner to cross the finish line isn't last place: it's running with a police escort.

1

Running From the Past

She's kneeling down in the grass to retie the laces on her sneaker, her long blonde ponytail hanging down her neck like a sleek ribbon. As she stands, her head turns slightly, peeking at my pale legs visible below the dark blue athletic shorts. Straightening, she turns to me with an amused smile blooming across her face and asks, "You're not shaving yet?"

I feel my cheeks burn. There are few things in life as traumatizing as the harsh humiliation of middle school mortification.

We were standing on the sidelines of the Junior Varsity Field, field hockey sticks in hand. It was the spring of 1993. Just a few months ago, William Jefferson Clinton was sworn in as President of the United States, unseating incumbent George H. W. Bush. That summer, I would somehow convince my mom to take me and my friend Katie to see the PG-13 film *Jurassic Park* at the movie theater and then convince my dad to let me see Meat Loaf in concert as part of his *Bat Out of Hell II* tour.

Given my taste in music and movies, my level of coolness was already questionable, but I was most decidedly not cool on that particular spring day, a few months before the end of sixth grade. No, I was an overweight eleven-year-old awkwardly holding a field hockey stick, sporting peach fuzz on my legs.

Situated behind the middle school, the JV field was smaller and less well-organized, and decidedly less permanent, than the varsity stadium that loomed in the distance. A patch of green grass with temporary white lines painted on it, lines that would inevitably need to be painted and repainted after enough gym classes stampeded over it. (I should say, as my peers stampeded over it. I saw the bright green grass of the JV field like a toxic waste dump and barely toed the lines and even then only when forced.)

The blonde and I were dressed alike, wearing dark blue shorts and a light blue shirt with the school district's logo—a large imposing ship— emblazoned over our hearts. I think her name was Jenny. But I only say that because I'm pretty sure all of the blondes of my graduating year were named Jenny. Well. All of the blondes except for me were named Jenny. Or Jennifer. Or Jen(n). This includes my best friend who is also, I might add, blonde. My little microcosm of classmates was a perfect illustration of the Most Popular Girl Names of 1981 *and* 1982.

Jill was ranked seventy-eighth on the list of popular girl names the year I was born. Thanks, Mom and Dad, for helping me fit in.

Right: so Jenny and I were dressed alike. Middle school was the first year my classmates and I got actual gym uniforms. Up until that point, physical education classes were held in whatever we happened to wear to school that day. But now we had graduated from the carefree days of grade school and entered the next chapter of our young lives: the tumultuous preteen years when acne, puberty, and hormones are still on the horizon, but creeping closer with each new school season. It was that age, precariously balanced between pretending to take Barbie and Ken on a date and actually going on a date, where we were all still attempting to define ourselves. We all wanted to set ourselves apart from our peers, but not so far apart that we risked being voted off the island of popularity and banished to *That Table* in the lunchroom.

So it was in the middle of all this adolescent angst that our school decided to add matching gym uniforms to the mix. Gym uniforms, I should add, that were neither flattering nor comfortable. My classmates and I also got lockers to keep them in, which meant there was a locker room that we changed in before and after class each day. As if wearing the same gym uniform as everyone else wasn't bad enough, we had to take them on and off in front of everyone else as well. And if that wasn't enough, both the shirt and the shorts had a spot to write our names. While I'm sure this was intended to help identify the owner if garments went missing, all I saw was my unathletic anonymity being whisked away.

That afternoon, after my exchange with Jenny, as soon as I got home from school, I locked myself in the bathroom and started digging in the cabinet beneath the sink, which was the home of my mom's stash of personal items related to the female constitution. Being an early bloomer, I was familiar with some of the items; but others, like the razor I eventually fished out with triumph, I was not.

Propping one leg on the lip of the tub, I rolled my pants up to my knee and applied the razor to my legs. That is, I took *only* a razor to my legs: in my haste to be like one of the cool girls with their smooth, shiny, peach-fuzz-free legs, I completely missed the part of the process that requires some kind of lubricant, like shaving cream or soap. Hell, even water would have been better than dragging that blade clean across my dry skin.

My legs burned for days, red and blotchy. But at least they were hair-free.

Because my own personal development far outpaced whatever limited elastic was included in the original gym shirt and shorts I was originally provided, the waistband on my pair of shorts eventually became tight over my burgeoning hips. One day after gym class, while I was walking back towards the school, one of the teachers came up to me and suggested I stop by her office after class to get a new (i.e. bigger) uniform.

See, I was always a little ahead on the developmental curve. I got my first real-life, grown-up bra in fifth grade. My mom tried to sell me on the whole YOU'RE A WOMAN NOW thing but my bullshit detector went off pretty early on that one and that same warning alarm reached near shrieking volumes when the stupid jackass who sat behind me in English class kept snapping my bra straps just because he could (and because he was a stupid jackass).

Having a matronly department store employee measure me in the fitting room of the local J. C. Penney while my mom waited outside was nowhere near as horrifying as having a *teacher* point out that I needed bigger clothes. Not only bigger clothes, but a bigger gym uniform. I mean, why couldn't it be a cute pair of jeans or something?

Looking back, I'm relatively certain these two events involving Jenny and my gym teacher happened on completely different days. They even might have occurred in completely different years. But in my muddled memory these two experiences have wound themselves tightly around each other, locked and knotted into one humiliating afternoon that symbolizes pretty much everything I loathed about forced physical education classes. Locker rooms, uniforms, body image, hormones. Really, it's amazing any preteen manages to make it to high school in one piece.

It *maybe* would have been tolerable if these situations had all spontaneously started to happen once puberty entered the scene, but for me it started way earlier when I was in elementary school, particularly during recess, that beloved hour of every school child. For my peers it meant an opportunity to escape the stifling pressures and education of the classroom to go run around for an hour. There were several elementary buildings in my school district, each complete with its own dedicated playground full of metal and concrete equipment, and faded squares of hopscotch, and jump rope, and basketballs. For my classmates, there seemed to be nothing worse than going down to the lunchroom and finding a sign that the playground was closed for the day due to inclement weather. The groans of disappointment would rumble over the paper cartons of chocolate milk and lukewarm chicken patty sandwiches. Nothing was worse than indoor recess.

Those weirdos, they loved that whole exerting energy thing.

But as for me? I mean, hello. We already had to run around in gym class. Why would you *voluntarily* do more of that? Especially when it's not even for a grade?

Recess, for me, was also an escape, but one that went into the secret worlds of the novels that lined the small wooden shelves of the school library. While I thought my peers were the weirdos for loving regular recess, I was the true weirdo who loved indoor recess because it meant I could spend the hour in the library. During outdoor recess, I was shuffled out onto the blacktop playground with the rest of my classmates. While they ran wild, I'd find a quiet corner along the brick wall of the building and bury myself in a book. My favorites were the *Scary Stories to Tell in the Dark* series, the macabre illustrations haunting my dreams. A few years ago they modernized—that is, sanitized—those illustrations and while the text remains the same, the stories are far less scary without those gruesome images.

(Along with being a total bookworm, there was also that incident in first or second grade where I was attempting to cross the monkey bars and my hands slipped, ending in a sprained ankle. Understandably, I was a little gun-shy around playground equipment after that.)

As a child, I was uncoordinated and unathletic. Even now, decades later, I'm only mildly less uncoordinated and only slightly more athletic. In the intervening years, between Jill-then and Jill-now, I also grew lazy, resisting pretty much any form of unnecessary physical activity. I mean, in a competition between me and a sloth, I'd probably win by a landslide. But, of course, such a competition would require either of us actually *doing* something which, well, y'know.

My mother, bless her soul, tried her hardest to combat my sedentary lifestyle, knowing full well it wasn't something I was going to decide to change on my own. Early on, she'd just push me out the door, tell me to get on my bicycle, and stay out for at least half an hour. Her intention, of course, was for me to actually ride the bike for half an hour. I, however, circumvented that by riding the five or so minutes it took to reach the local park, and preceded to hang out there for twenty minutes, and then rode my bike back home.

I felt no guilt about this. After all, I was honoring my mother's intention, if not abiding by its spirit. If nothing else, at least I was spending that time outside, instead of holed up in my bedroom.

Eventually she either caught on to my ruse or simply decided more drastic measures were needed. Much to my dismay, these drastic measures were ones that could be measured at home.

With the exercise bike living in our basement, although it technically belonged to my dad, who frequently used it, my mom saw a golden opportunity. I would ride that bike. Not only would I ride that bike, I was expected to keep track of how many minutes I rode and report back to her.

There was also a carrot. Oh yes: eventually it got to the point where my mother decided her only recourse was to bribe me and she knew just the way to do it.

My musical choices have always been a little, shall we say, questionable for my age. I straddle that generation between X and Millennials, and while I grew up in the era of New Kids on the Block, I spent most of my childhood absorbing the classic rock roots of my father. To this day, I can't tell you a single song that NKOTB or Boyz II Men ever sang, but I can sing the entire lyrics to Billy Joel's "We Didn't Start the Fire" and explain the historical and cultural significance of Crosby, Stills, Nash & Young's "Ohio." Before finally owning a personal copy on CD, I wore out my dad's cassette tape of Pink Floyd's *The Dark Side of the Moon* and borrowed-with-no-intention-of-returning countless Led Zeppelin albums.

As if that didn't make me different enough, I also developed a strong attraction to the theatre. Mixed in with all of those hard rock musicians, there was a healthy dose of Broadway show tunes, often accompanied with father-daughter dates to Playhouse Square in downtown Cleveland to see live performances. Andrew Lloyd Webber was my gateway drug but my love soon progressed to Sondheim and Schwartz among other greats.

So it was in the mid-1990s, when half of my female friends were freaking out about the latest boy band to hit the block and the other half of my female friends were still mourning the death of Kurt Cobain,

I was glued to my television the night of Barbra Streisand's triumphant return to the stage with her first concert in almost thirty years.

When the live, double-CD album *Barbra: The Concert* was released in late 1994, I simply *had* to have it the same way my friends *had* to have their first row seats to the 98 Degrees concert so they could gawk over Cincinnatians Nick and Drew Lachey up close and in person. I wasn't babysitting neighborhood kids quite yet so my funds were limited to the small weekly allowance I got for doing chores around the house.

In my love for Barbra, my mom saw an opportunity and struck a deal: if I logged a certain amount of hours on that exercise bike, she and my dad would buy me the album as a reward. I already had a slight aversion to bikes, even indoor ones—thanks to a good chunk of my summers spent being told to go riding—but I also really, really wanted that album.

I can't for the life of me remember exactly how many hours I needed to clock in to earn the CD, but every day after school I'd go downstairs and I'd pedal my little heart out. I wasn't doing it for enjoyment or for exercise. I don't even think the fact that I was doing something good for my body even crossed my mind. I was down there working out for one reason and one reason only. As soon as I had that album in my hands, I never got on that bike again.

Given my absolute animosity towards athletics of any kind, it probably goes without say that I still loathed gym class by the time I got to high school. If anything, I probably hated it *more*, if that's even possible. Hell, I hated gym class more than I hated math class, which is certainly saying something considering my strong aversion to arithmetic throughout middle school and high school. (This came back to haunt me when I decided to get my master's in Library and Information Science and had to take the GRE. My prep work consisted of vocabulary words and focusing on the English portion since I knew there was no way in hell I was going to do well on the Math section, so I might as well put my energy into working on the one area I knew I could improve on. Later, as a professional adult, I interviewed for a job at a college that required taking an evaluation test. I knew I aced the English portion but I distinctly remember telling friends and family, "If I don't get that position because of stupid fractions, I'm going to be so pissed." Either my math skills aren't as horrible as I think or I guessed well, because I did get the job.)

Now, the only thing that made high school gym class slightly more tolerable than middle school is that we were given options. No longer did our gym teachers decide for us what activity we were going to do that week. No more were we told we *had* to play soccer or we *had* to play basketball. Nope, we were now independent! and capable! and self-sufficient! young adults! Soon we would be driving and voting for the next president.

Perhaps realizing that we were only a few years away from becoming legal adults, our gym teachers allowed some flexibility in the schedule by presenting choices at the beginning of the week: one option would be on the more athletic side like soccer or basketball, while the other option was something a little more on the non-traditional side.

In high school, class schedules were somewhat random, and obviously depended entirely on what classes I took. This meant there was no real way to guarantee I'd have lunch with friends and thus get to commiserate about how much we hated baseball. I always seemed to luck out by having at least one or two friends in my gym class and we had an unspoken agreement between us that when presented with options we would always, always pick the least athletic one.

This variety meant that the majority of my high school physical education curriculum was comprised of multiple weeks of weight training on the same big industrial machines used by the varsity football team, learning just how *exactly* to score a bowling game by hand, and at least one memorable week of ping pong in which my friends and I played our own onomatopoeia version of ping pong. (This specialized version stipulated that each time we hit the ball we would shout a word like *POW!* or *ZAP!*, imagining bright graphics like those from the old Batman television show.)

But for all the awesomeness that came with having choices like that in gym, there was one thing that we could never, ever get out of doing.

The Annual Mile.

Oh, the mile. Otherwise known as 5,280 feet of torture for awkward teenagers everywhere. It was only four measly laps around the track out back behind the school, but for me they might as well have been forty laps.

The thing is, I couldn't run. Not, I didn't want to. Not, I didn't like to (well, I mean, I didn't like to then). Quite honestly, I could not for the life of me run for more than a couple yards without wanting to pass out. Between the inability to breathe and the fact that my legs felt like lead, there was certainly nothing enjoyable about running. I got hot. I got sweaty. I hurt, all over. *WHY WOULD PEOPLE VOLUNTARILY PUT THEIR BODIES THROUGH THIS*? It was like being in a torture chamber without there being any bizarre spikes jutting out from the wall. From this experience, I didn't really understand the point of running for exercise, let alone entertainment. Running for any reason other than being chased by a hungry bear was a completely foreign concept to me.

As a child of the 1980s, I was introduced to a wide range of pop culture icons that still permeate our culture today. One of these in particular stuck with me, to the point that I take great delight in knowing that my birthday is the same date as the Hill Valley High "Enchantment Under the Sea" Dance of *Back to the Future* fame. I didn't start driving until I was nineteen, but at sixteen, man oh man did I want a DeLorean. Never mind the fact that it would just be a boring car and not a time machine, but man I would have looked so *cool* driving one of those things around.

("Cool" in this context might be subjective, but I proudly let my geek flag fly.)

In the third and final installment of the *Back to the Future* trilogy, there is a scene where Marty and Doc Brown are hanging out in a saloon in the Old West, trying to figure out how to, uh, get, y'know, back to the future. In a rare moment of consequence ignoring, Doc is explaining to some old cowboys in the saloon about technology in the future, including the fact that we no longer use horses for transportation because we have automobiles. So, the skeptical denizens of the past ask, if everyone has one of these automobile things, do people still even walk or run in the future?

"Of course we run," Doc Brown tells them. "But for recreation; for fun."

One of the cowboys scoffs. "Run for fun? What the hell kind of fun is that?"

Preach, you old cowboy you.

~~~

I graduated from high school almost twenty years ago, so maybe it's for that reason that I sincerely am unable to remember exactly how often we met for gym class. That, or I just completely blocked it all out, which is also a very fair guess, too.

Anyway, it would have been maybe tolerable had the Annual Mile been only a mile. Or, well, I guess, only one day. But it wasn't, because our class met more than once a week and so the gym needed to find a way to stretch the Annual Mile and make it last for several class periods. This meant that in the days leading up to Mile Day, we were taken on short runs around the school. Sometimes we'd run one or two laps on the track, other times they'd take us out across the fields used by the cross country team. Either way, there was lots of running before we actually ran the Mile.

Now, of course, I understand that this is what we fancy runners tend to call "training." Just like you don't wake up one morning and decide to go run a half marathon, in Hudson High School, unless you were on the track team, chances were you weren't regularly running any distance even close to a mile. These days I know that following an appropriate training plan is one of the things that keeps us runners relatively injury free on race day, and our gym teachers were being judicious in their decision to provide us with a training regimen in the weeks leading up to the actual running of the Mile.

But I didn't know that back then. All I knew was that it was more running that I didn't want to do.

Before I go any further I should make one thing absolutely clear: *I never—not once—ever ran the Mile in school.* Never ever. I didn't run it in middle school and I definitely didn't run it in high school.

Yes siree, I was a walker. Walking was easy. Walking was something I did every day. After all, I walked around the school to get to class.

Friday nights during the fall I marched (a close cousin to walking) as a member of the Hudson High School "Swing" Marching Band. Walking I could do forever, unlike running which I could only manage for very, very short distances or perhaps if I was in fear for my life.

Naturally, the gym teachers would get frustrated by me and classmates like myself. Every year, there were the runners—the *real* runners— out there on the track, completing their mile in five or six minutes. I was only just starting my second lap at that point. For four Annual Miles in a row, I didn't even try and pretend to pick up my pace when I was crossing in front of the teacher with the stop watch; I just kept my slow and steady twenty-minute-mile walking pace. The teachers would try and encourage me to gain a little speed and suggest I walk the straight lengths of the track and run the curves.

Just try, they'd say.

So I would. For maybe a lap, maybe less. But then I went back to my walking.

Running made me uncomfortable. In the act, I felt ungainly, lumbering around the track in front of all of my classmates. I was exposed and vulnerable. As someone who has always been on the heavier side, I knew I didn't look like a runner, and when you're in high school looks count for everything. Runners are lean and lithe. Runners are athletic with thick calves that carry them quickly across finish lines. Runners are built for speed.

I looked like a walker. So, I walked.

Year after year. Mile after mile. Four laps around that track.

My gym teachers tolerated my walking because they obviously had no way of physically forcing me to run, but it was clear they wanted me to run. Alternative methods like walking weren't just frowned upon, they weren't even discussed. Nope, all the students were just expected to run, and run well, and run fast and, worst yet, run for a grade.

To be fair, the grade given was mostly a participation thing where as long as a student showed up and did something they were given an A, but compulsory running is a very different experience than voluntary running.

The problem wasn't the grading of the Annual Mile. The problem was treating all students as if they are members of the track team, expressing the sentiment that running is no big deal, and if you think it is a big deal, then there is something wrong with you. Bottom line, it meant that if you couldn't run fast, then there is something wrong with you. If you can't keep up, then there is something wrong with you. And if you need to walk or are having trouble breathing, then there is really something wrong with you.

For a physical education class, there was very little education related to running. We were set loose on the track and expected to just run without any discussion about healthy habits such as the benefits of run-walk intervals or how to find the right pace. Nope, we were just supposed to run, and if we couldn't compete with the 5- and 6-minute mile averages of the track team then we should be grateful for that participation grade because we'd be failing otherwise.

But in the end, it's all okay because I still managed to graduate, so in all reality gym class really isn't the end all be all class they often make it out to be.

2

One Foot in Front of the Other

Jillian Michaels is yelling, her aggressive voice filling my living room. On my television screen, that is. Jillian Michaels is yelling on my television screen to the newest group of recruits who have been rescued from their gluttonous lifestyles in middle America and swept away to glamorous California, home of the California avocado and the California sushi roll, which is made with avocado, and probably other Californian foods that sound like they can only be consumed in a sunny spa with a glass of sparkling water on the side, by the extravagantly glamorous and wealthy.

(Did you know that all Hass avocados can trace their ancestral roots and actual roots to the same avocado tree that was planted by Randolph Hass in California in 1926? She's literally the Mother Tree of all Hass avocados. I sort of secretly hope Randolph named her Eve.)

So. Jillian Michaels is yelling at the contestants, and Bob Harper is doing his Zen Master thing on the yoga mat, and I'm on the couch for the second weekend in a row binge-watching *The Biggest Loser*.

The irony of this situation is not lost on me.

My feelings for this particular reality show ebb and flow, not unlike the waistline of a yo-yo dieter. As a woman who has spent her entire life as "fat," I connect with the journeys of the men and women on the show in a very visceral way. I *understand* them. I understand what drives them to drive to the twenty-four-hour McDonald's at two o'clock in the morning for a twenty-piece McNugget and a large side of fries. I understand how they can consume 3,000 calories in a single meal and still be hungry an hour later. I understand their reluctance to join a gym and risk making an ass of themselves in front of all the regulars.

And most of all, I really understand their aversion to the dreaded treadmill.

I understand all of this because I spent much of my adult life being one of those people. I understand them because more than once I'd head to the local fast food joint several times a day, snarfing down an extra-large value meal in front of the television while watching other people work out.

Growing up, I'd been a pretty chubby kid and so clothes shopping was the absolute worst. Now that we live in an age of positive body love, I enjoy needing to go out and buy a new dress or work clothes, but in the mid-1990s the majority of designers were loathe to make garments for fat people. Because obviously fat people deserve to wear ugly clothes as punishment for being fat. (Granted, some designers still don't like fat people wearing their label, but there are less of them these days and, even better, more designers who design specifically for those on the larger side of the size spectrum.)

When you're sixteen years old, there is literally nothing more mortifying than needing to shop in the Women's Department of the store. I was basically shopping at the same stores as my mom, which did very little for both my self-esteem and sense of style. And prom dresses? Bitch, please. While all of my other friends could go spend an afternoon at the mall trying on a wide variety of fancy dresses, my size sixteen prom dress was actually a bridesmaid dress that had to be ordered from a *catalog*. I'm not even talking about online shopping, either. Oh no, this was the kind of paper catalog that showed up in the mail and required calling the 1-800 number to place your order.

Starting in my teenage years and going up through my late

twenties, I basically wore my age. This means that by the time I got to be twenty-nine, I was wearing a size twenty-eight pair of jeans and tipped the scales at 311 pounds.

Truthfully, I didn't even really know how much I weighed because the analog scale that I owned didn't go up that high. It capped out at 250 or something, and I could just see that little red dial pushing against the side of the window, confused and frustrated by its inability to register the information.

I don't know if I can verbally express what it means to be so heavy that you literally outweigh your scale's capabilities. Like, seriously. Just think about that for a second, okay? A scale has a pretty basic function. Really, it only has one function: to display the weight of the item on it, whether it's ounces of food or pounds of people. That's it. That is the scale's only job, and I had gotten so big, I put my scale out of work.

I not only had to go out and buy a brand new scale but I also didn't have the luxury of picking whatever scale caught my fancy. I had to read the boxes carefully to make sure that I bought one that would be able to measure what I was bringing to the table.

Of course, my table looked like the local all-you-can-eat buffet, so there wasn't much room left for anything but dessert (because, duh, there's always room for dessert). What I thought I needed was a new scale but what I *really* needed was someone to wake me the fuck up.

So one morning, I woke up to an email from my younger sister Amy, who was very concerned about my weight and the overall impact it would have on my health. My family had attempted to have similar conversations with me in the past and I always got incredibly defensive, so I think Amy was prepared for the same kind of reaction this time around.

Instead, I knew that my weight had reached a critical junction and that she and the rest of my family were right. I needed to do something and I needed to do something now, so soon after I joined Weight Watchers.

I'd been on Weight Watchers for a year, and was down about fifty pounds or so when I found myself totally engrossed in watching *The*

Biggest Loser. Almost all of the weight I had lost thus far was because of a shift in my diet and food choices, not my activity level. I was still pretty much as lazy as always.

My feelings for this show are complicated because I do sympathize and empathize and identify with the contestants. But as a woman who has spent her entire life trying to lose weight, taking advantage of a variety of means and methods through which to do so, I really loathe the drastic techniques utilized by *The Biggest Loser* and the unrealistic expectations it sets up, especially for contestants. In most any other situation where losing weight was the goal, two or three pounds in a single week would be tremendous and certainly worth celebrating. Instead, because of the competitive nature of the show, as well as the amount of time dedicated to exercise each day, two or three pounds in a week is seen as a failure and the contestants come away feeling bad about themselves, as though they haven't done enough work.

But I also recognize that the show can provide a certain level of motivation. I should know, because watching those men and women running on the treadmill, men and women who weighed a good 100 or 200 pounds more than I did at that moment in time, triggered something inside of me. I found myself watching them with a sense of wonder and awe. All I wanted to do was get up and move.

So I did the only thing I could think to do: I decided to go for a run.

I will totally appreciate if this is the point in my story where you're giving me a bit of side-eye, just a little bit confused. After all, just a chapter ago I was all, *I HATE RUNNING! RUNNING IS THE WORST!* and now all of a sudden I'm all, *LET'S GO RUNNING! YAY RUNNING!*

Honestly, I have no idea where the desire to run came from because, trust me, never before in my entire life had I ever felt this pull to go for a run. That's really what it was like, though, a pull. Some outside force grabbing hold and tugging me along. It was just some little voice in the back of my head that bubbled up all of a sudden, and I decided it was better to just go with it and listen to that voice instead of waiting for some other voice in my head that would tell me this was the most ridiculous idea ever.

Since returning to Northeast Ohio after graduate school and moving to Cleveland, I'd lived in a converted warehouse near downtown. It's an industrial neighborhood lacking in close proximity to parks and public green space and sidewalks—basically all things crucial to a good outdoor run. Thankfully, it's since changed in the near decade that I've been here, but at the time when that little voice told me to get up and run, outside wasn't the most ideal. It was also early February, which is a tenuous time when you're living in a temperate climate.

In the lobby of my building is a small little room that has been converted to a mini gym for the residents, including an elliptical, some strength training equipment, and, yes, a treadmill. Not that I'd ever really used any of the machines.

After spending most of the day horizontal on my couch, I suddenly sat up and turned the television off, the episode only half over. Those contestants were running on that treadmill with speeds of 7 mph, which is like an 8-minute mile pace. Sure, because of their size, limited mobility, and unfamiliarity with exercise they could maybe only maintain that pace for a minute or so but that's far faster and longer than I'd ever run before. Even in high school when I agreed to run the straight lanes and walk the curves of the track, I certainly wasn't putting in any kind of real effort. I was doing the bare minimum of what it would take to get my gym teachers to stop nagging me so I could receive a passing grade.

I can claim that I can't run all I like, and I can claim I don't like running, but can I really say that either of those statements are fact when I've never really given running a good old-fashioned, honest try?

This may come as no surprise if you gotten this far, but I'm someone with lots of opinions. I know what I like and I know what I don't. But I don't come to those opinions blindly or from a biased perspective. I can tell you beyond a shadow of a doubt that I do not like the writing of Joyce Carol Oates. But I can also back that up by telling you that I have attempted to read at least half a dozen of her novels and quit halfway through each and every one of them. So, yes, when I say I do not like the writing of Joyce Carol Oates, I firmly say this with my own anecdotal evidence to back it up.

But when it came to running, my anecdotal evidence was pretty much nonexistent, because, honestly, I'd never really run. But being a mature adult means that sometimes you realize that things you hated when you were younger are things you love as an adult, if you're just willing to give them a second chance.

Kind of like Brussels sprouts.

Now during my teenage years, my dad would go on and off the Atkins Diet plan, only he wouldn't tell my mom, who was our de facto meal planner. She'd only know he was "on" plan when he would decline whatever dinner she had made that night and just eat a big bowl of Brussels sprouts for dinner. Brussels sprouts weren't something my family really ever ate when I was growing up, and so my only real exposure was sitting there at the table with my dad and his bowl of steamed sprouts. Their smell was so pungent and funky that from a young age, I pretty much swore them off and anytime anyone would serve me Brussels sprouts I had a weird Pavlovian gag reflex response.

Then one day my friend Lauren invited me over for dinner. A vegan, Lauren made me this fantastic meal that included the dreaded Brussels sprouts as a side dish. Not wanting to be an ungracious guest, I took a small bite and was delighted to discover I found them quite delicious, and cleaned my whole plate. She hadn't really done anything fancy to them, shredded them and maybe roasted them in the oven. But whatever she did, they trumped whatever bad memory I had of Brussels sprouts from my youth.

Turns out, running is kind of like the Brussels sprouts of athletics. It really is just a matter of how they are served.

But, unlike unsavory vegetables, athletics requires equipment. For instance, running requires running shoes.

My first position as a professional librarian after graduate school was at a minimum security prison on the far west side of Cleveland. My first professional day at said job was spent not at the prison, but off-site at an unarmed self-defense class where I got to interact with some of my new colleagues by pretending to break up prison fights and put handcuffs on the "inmates." I was instructed to show up dressed to work out. The clothes portion of that was easy—despite rarely exercising I had enough yoga pants to open up my own yoga studio, but I was forced to go out and buy appropriate shoes. I went to Walmart per their website and bought the cheapest pair of tennis shoes they had in my size. I wore them to that unarmed self-defense class before I started and to the annual orientation a year later, and then put them securely back in my closet, where they sat collecting dust until that fateful day in February 2012.

After silencing Jillian Michaels with the remote, I went into my bedroom and started digging through my closet. I pulled out a pair of yoga pants, a random tee shirt, and my tennis shoes. I laced the shoes up, grabbed my iPhone and headphones, and headed downstairs to the mini gym.

Stepping on the treadmill, I decided trying to recreate what happened in *The Biggest Loser* gym was probably not the smartest nor safest idea, and decided to try slow-paced intervals instead.

I started with 30:90 intervals, which meant I walked for 30 seconds and ran for 90 seconds on a treadmill set at 3 mph. One foot in front of the other, walk then run then walk. During the running intervals the pace of the treadmill stayed the same, I just picked up my feet and speed a bit more. I kept those intervals up for 20 minutes and by the end I had gone a complete mile.

I hated every single second of those twenty minutes. My body hurt, moving muscles that hadn't been moved in such a way in years, if ever.

But after? Oh, after I felt powerful and strong. It was hard work but worth it.

Turns out, running wasn't so bad after all.

I decided, though, that if I was going to give this whole running thing a try I needed a more structured plan. I am someone who likes structure, who likes to have a concrete set of instructions to follow. It's probably one reason why these days I absolutely love training for a race.

After doing a little bit of research about starting to run online, I decided to try the Couch to 5K plan, which is a pretty popular option for beginners. For someone who has done zero running before, it really does take you from the Couch to running a 5K distance of 3.1 miles. It operates on intervals, basically what I was already doing but in a more structured way. The plan has runners initially begin by walking more than they run, but as they progress through the program, those intervals swap until they are completely running without walking breaks. It lasts nine weeks and you only have to do it three times a week, with the runs being 20 to 30 minutes in length.

Trying to pay attention to intervals while on a treadmill is pretty much impossible. For one thing, I can't cover up the treadmill dashboard with my towel to hide the distance because I have to be able to watch the clock. For another thing, having to constantly watch the clock means I can't go into that really awesome running zone. The one where I tune out the world around me and just do my thing. The not being able to cover up the dashboard is more annoying than anything else; I just hate looking down at the mileage and seeing I haven't gone nearly as far as I feel like I have. But not getting into the zone is frustrating and can cause a run to turn into a bad one.

So I did that one thing I never, ever do: I actually paid money for an app on my phone.

The C25K app is set up just like the information on the website, only instead of having to constantly watch the clock to see if you should be running or walking, there is a voice that tells you when to run and when to walk. That way all I had to do was speed up during the running parts and slow down during the walking parts *and* I could still cover up the dashboard so I didn't have to see those stupid little dots moving around a big electronic loop, slowly marking off a mile.

There are three "trainers" to choose from: one is modeled after a military sergeant, one is a nice encouraging female, and one is more of a hard-core female who reminded me quite a lot of a certain reality television trainer.

Guess which one I chose.

I mean, if I can't have the actual Jillian Michaels yelling at me I might as well have some digital off-brand copy of her yelling at me, amirite?

At the time I started running, my work schedule was weird. And by "weird," I mean annoying. And by "annoying," I mean I was working twelve hour days, Monday through Thursday. Four days a week, I'd work 9 a.m. until 9 p.m. and because I lived a good forty-five minutes away in summer (and closer to an hour in winter), I'd leave the house at about 8 a.m. and not get home until close to 10 p.m.

Apparently my masochistic side decided it needed more pain, so I added in after work runs on Monday and Wednesday evenings.

Looking back, I'm not sure why I settled on evening runs in the beginning, especially considering how late at night I was getting on the treadmill. But clearly it made sense at the time. Considering even now, years later, I pretty much want to hibernate every morning in winter, I suspect that was part of my reasoning back then, too. I am a total freeze baby, and this is Cleveland, and it's *cold* in the mornings during winter. Really cold. Like, I can't even, kind of cold. The kind of cold that can only be combatted by burrowing deep, deep under layers and layers of blankets and two cats.

The only upside to this schedule was that I had three-day weekends every weekend. Having every Friday off was really glorious just from a sleeping in on a cold morning perspective, but it also meant that I could go running in the morning.

My progress through the C25K app was going smoothly, and while the app allows you to repeat a week of exercises if you didn't feel quite ready to move to the next week, I continued to move ahead week after week after week. As the weeks melted into each other, so, too, did the snow outside. Soon, running indoors on the treadmill held less appeal. It was just so *boring*. It had always been boring, but it was better than the alternative of bundling up, and I certainly didn't have appropriate outdoor winter running apparel hanging in my closet. With the change of seasons, however, I was in a position to take my legs off the machine and into the great, big world.

I mean, really. How different could it be to run outside?

The thing is, I *know* the answer to that question. This one I actually had anecdotal evidence to back up and I'm not even talking about those four laps around the track out back behind my high school.

Many, many years ago my friend Lisa was celebrating a birthday at a roller skating rink. Now while I say many years ago, Lisa was still in her late twenties at this point. Being a woman who celebrated turning twenty-nine with a Hannah Montana themed party, I'm hardly in a position to judge. The thing is, I never learned how to roller skate. My version of "skating" involves planting one foot and using the other foot to maneuver. It's some weird fusion between roller skating and skateboarding. I just had never learned the proper technique of alternating your feet on roller skates.

As such, I spent much of the skating party on the sidelines watching friends, but it was okay because, lemme tell ya, roller skating rinks make for fascinating people-watching.

After hours watching people skate, I decided I wanted to learn how to skate. I've always had this vision of being a badass roller derby girl (never mind the fact that I can't actually skate) and this seemed like an opportunity to finally learn. As luck would have it, I was at a thrift store that weekend and came across a pair of *rollerblades*. True, it's not quite the same thing, but that's what the thrift store had, so that's what I was buying.

The foyer and dining room of my apartment are hardwood and I actually spent a couple days just skating around my apartment on the hardwood floor, getting used to the feel and movement of being on the skates.

A few nights later, I decided to take the rollerblades outside. After all, how different could it be from skating around my apartment?

I'll spare you the suspense: it's different. Very different.

Keep in mind, I live in an industrial area in a major metropolitan city. At the time, it was also a neglected area of the city. Don't get me wrong, I love my neighborhood. I love living among the noisy city streets and bumping right up against the Cuyahoga. I don't even mind being woken up by the sounds of ships passing in the night. But we are not high on the priority list of the City of Cleveland when it comes to maintenance. Sidewalks, in particular, are uneven. Quite uneven.

To the point that I fell on my ass as soon as I was out the door.

My balance has always been a little unstable so stick some wheels on my feet and, well, shit's about to get real. In my apartment I had the option of using a hand to catch myself against a chair or a table or a wall if necessary. Such luxuries are not afforded in the great, big, wide world which is why it is advised that those partaking in such activities should wear these newfangled gadgets called knee and elbow pads, neither of which I had, I might add.

Never one to be deterred by a single fall, I crawled to a nearby electric pole and braced myself against it as I hoisted my fat ass back up onto the rollerblades.

I made it half a city block before falling on my ass again. Only this time I didn't just fall on my ass and wound my pride: *I broke my elbow.*

What kind of late twentysomething breaks a bone attempting to relive some naive dream to be a fucking roller derby girl?

I do. Me. This one right here. I'm that kind of girl.

So I should have known better than to just assume that going from the comfort of a temperature-controlled gym to the brave outdoors would be an easy transition.

For one thing, temperature is not the only thing controlled when you're running inside on a treadmill. Your pace is, too: there is a belt that maintains a predetermined speed which means *you* maintain a predetermined speed. Maintaining the exact same speed over a long distance is *hard*, yo. Most runners aim for and admire other runners who have negative splits, runners who successfully get faster with each mile. Me, though, I have great respect for the pacers. Those runners who sometimes carry signs on wooden sticks with the expected finish time so those in the pack know who to keep up with if they are looking to finish a half or full marathon in a certain time. Those pacers are hard-core and have the ability to keep a steady and constant pace for the duration of an entire race. They are like the human equivalent of a treadmill.

All those weeks on the treadmill, I never paid any attention to the data. I ran when my Couch to 5K app told me I should run, and I walked when it told me I should walk, and I stopped when the daily program stopped.

Outside, though, I not only had the Couch to 5K app, I had the option of using other apps, too. Ones that utilized a GPS to track distance and pace in a real-world context and not just the drumming of a belt around a loop.

Running through that crisp air that hovered between the briskness of winter and the warm of seasons to come, I ran around my neighborhood, up and down the streets, following the natural curve of the Cuyahoga. My body was challenged as it adapted to the new environment around me. I had to watch for cars and approach intersections with caution. About halfway through that initial outdoor run, I paused briefly on the sidewalk and a passing white car honked. When I looked up, the driver was giving me a thumbs-up sign.

That was my first introduction to the supportive community that is running.

At the end of my run I checked the app on my phone that had been tracking my distance and speed to see how long it had taken me to run that first full mile.

Sixteen minutes.

Being a new runner, I didn't think anything of it. Okay, so it took me sixteen minutes to run a mile. It's certainly faster than the twenty-plus it took me to walk it in high school.

Not being a runner, not coming from a running family, and not having any previous exposure to the sport, I didn't really know what made one fast or slow. I didn't know that things like 5- and 6-minute miles existed in mortal men but even if I had, I don't know if it would have made any difference in my positive attitude towards my own speed. I was still so enraptured with the idea that I was *running* that how fast or slow I was running didn't really seem to matter. Without anyone else to compare my own progress to, I just did my own thing.

But I soon realized that if I was going to keep doing my own thing then I really needed to do it in a pair of appropriate shoes. The very basic pair of athletic shoes I had purchased years ago at a big-box store got the job done up until this point, but if I was *serious* about this and going to be a *serious* runner and do *serious* runner things then I needed a serious pair of shoes.

Running as an activity is pretty inexpensive. While special gear exists and exists in abundance—heart rate monitors, GPS watches, pouches or arm sleeves for your phone, etc.—none of it is necessary to be a runner. You can buy fancy patterned running tights and celebrity-endorsed athletic tops, but you can just as easily be a successful runner wearing a pair of shorts you found on the cheap and a ratty t-shirt you pulled out of your closet.

Know what's not inexpensive? Decent running shoes.

But if you're a serious runner and want to do serious runner things, decent running shoes are a necessity. Wearing the wrong pair of shoes can lead to injury, which can lead to your running career ending before it even begins. While dropping a couple hundred dollars on a pair of shoes that you'll inevitably need to replace every few months (depending on how often you run) might seem overly expensive, that couple hundred is way cheaper than any hospital bills that may pop up after a serious running injury.

When I started, I naively thought all running shoes were created equal. Alas, they are not, mostly because not all runners and feet are created equal. Also, not all stores that sell running shoes are created equal either.

Over lunch with my friend Staci one weekend, I was talking about a need for new running shoes when she mentioned she used to work at a specialty running store. "They'll look at your feet and find you a pair of shoes that fits the way you run." Big-box athletic stores, she explained, won't do that. In terms of selling general sports equipment, they are good at their job. But when it comes to something as individual and intimate as running shoes, they are a bit out of their depth because it isn't their sole focus. Specialty running stores specialize in merchandise specifically for runners and their employees are trained in helping runners find the right running shoe. The kind of running shoe that will minimize risk of injury and work with my feet, not against them.

True to Staci's word, my old shoes got a thorough examination as the employee at Cleveland Running Company looked at the wear and tear pattern my running stride had left behind. Then my feet got an equally detailed analysis, as the sales clerk looked at the arch and other things completely unseen to my naked eye. From underneath the bench she pulled a metal measurement device out and measured my foot.

After taking it all in, she went to the wall of shoes, pulled a pair down, and handed them to me. I tried on the first pair and flexed my feet a little, adjusting to the fit. My idea of shoes for any sort of sport was as a heavy, solid thing. These were so light and airy, they felt like slippers. There was no way I could possibly *run* in these, which is what I told her when she asked how they fit.

With a nod, she went back to the wall and pulled another pair of shoes down, a pair that looked much more like what I had in mind.

I laced up the shoes and stood up, bouncing on my heels a little. Eyeing my feet closely, she asked how they felt.

"Much better," I answered.

She nodded. "Good," she said, nodding towards the door at the front of the store. "You can go outside if you want to try them out."

I furrowed my brow. "Outside?"

"Sure," she said. "You can just run up and down out on the sidewalk."

Still perplexed, I continued to just stand there.

A small smile appeared. "It's okay, I promise. You need to be able to try them out."

Even though she had given me the go ahead, and even though this was clearly something real runners did all the time, I pushed open the door with trepidation and stepped outside wearing the shoes. It felt so *wrong* to wear fancy expensive shoes I hadn't paid for outside. And then to actually, y'know, go running in them outside.

But run I did. The sidewalk outside was covered by an awning and I did a short jog up the block, past the other stores in the shopping strip, then turned around and came back.

Walking back inside, I gave her a single nod and said, "I'll take them."

With that single purchase, I had made a decision. Running shoes are not cheap, not by any stretch of the imagination, and by putting my money where my mouth was, I had committed to seeing this through.

I was already a runner. A real runner. But with that purchase of shoes, I now actually felt like one.

~~~

As much as I talk about living in a very industrial section of Cleveland, I am still blessed to live in a city that takes pride in providing its residents with lots of public green spaces. The Cleveland Metroparks encompass over 20,000 acres of networked parks that include rivers, walking and biking trails, education centers, golf courses . . . pretty much anything and everything you could think of to fit into 20,000 acres of open public space.

From my apartment, the closest of these parks is Edgewater Beach, situated on the near West Side of the city. Bumping up against Lake Erie, the park offers magnificent views of both downtown and the coast. A multilevel park, the lower level has the actual beach and a big paved loop that is almost exactly one mile around. Near the parking lot, the loop branches off to a quarter-mile hill that takes runners and walkers up to the upper level which has its own loop that is about half a mile around.

When I first moved to Cleveland, I had a limited view of how much this city had to offer. Technically I live downtown, although because I live on the West Side of the Cuyahoga, I consider myself a West Sider. Like many cities with delineated neighborhoods, there is a fierce loyalty when it comes to the East Side versus West Side conversation amongst residents. Even now, seven years after moving back, I still feel like I need a passport to visit the East Side of the city.

My friends lived in a nearby neighborhood, Tremont, with another neighborhood, Ohio City, sandwiched between us, so, for the most part, these were the two neighborhoods I visited regularly. Rarely did I venture to the suburbs, even those on the West Side, no matter how close I was to the city limits. This meant that Edgewater Park, which is situated roughly halfway between my apartment and the city of Lakewood, was virtually unknown territory to me.

Here's the thing: once you run outside, it's really hard to go back to running inside. Especially when you don't have to. Once I started not only running outside but running in the morning, I suddenly would spend all day at my job dreading having to get on the treadmill after work. Morning running is my mojo. I not only had those endorphins with me all day long, but when I got home from work I was done for the evening. I could just decompress from the day and relax. Eventually I took advantage of the fact that the C25K program is flexible and moved my running schedule around a little bit. Instead of running twice a week after work and Friday mornings, I now was going to run Wednesday mornings before work on the treadmill, and Friday and Sunday mornings outside.

I had been running outside in my neighborhood for a couple weeks when one morning I woke up and decided I wanted to try running in the park. It was a gorgeous day and I had the whole morning ahead of me. More than anything, I wanted a change of scenery.

After parking my car, I walked across the small parking lot and kept walking across the loop to the beach. The waves of Lake Erie lapped up against the sand and I just took a moment to breathe in the serene scene in front of me. I plugged my earbuds in, the music thumping through, and set off on a short two-mile run.

Because it was a weekday morning and most people were at work, I pretty much had the entire park to myself except for a few retirees walking their dogs. For two miles, two turns around that main loop, I just ran and ran and ran. I didn't have to watch for cars or worry about oncoming traffic. I didn't have to stop at intersections and wait to make sure it was safe to cross. The retirees and I would exchange brief nods and smiles as we passed each other but other than those small exchanges, I was completely on my own and in my own head.

It was nothing short of glorious.

The body is an amazing machine capable of achieving so much, physically. Running indoors on the treadmill always made me feel strong because I was doing something I'd never done before, but running outdoors and having the ability and mental space to really tap in and just zone out and only focus on my run made me feel ready to conquer the world.

I was a runner. It didn't matter how fast—or, in my case, how slow—I went. It didn't matter how long it took me to run those two miles because *I ran those two miles.*

After that, I turned to the treadmill only out of desperation and spent all week looking forward to those outdoor runs at Edgewater. I was still making my way through the Couch to 5K app, running three times a week, my walking intervals getting shorter and shorter with each run.

So, this one particular Friday I was up earlier than normal and found myself anxiously waiting for the initial glimmer of a pink sunrise over the downtown horizon. The air was still cool enough to require an extra layer of clothing, but as soon as it was light enough, I grabbed my gear and headed to Edgewater Park for my run.

My plan was an easy two miles, which was twice around the main big loop at the park. Two easy, peasy miles. With the bright rays of sun bouncing off the surface of Lake Erie, I cued up my running playlist on my phone and off I went.

As I came up to the crest of the loop on my second lap I realized I didn't want to stop. I felt like I was flying, as if wings had sprouted from the blades of my shoulders, carrying me back and forth across the park. Instead of being tired, my legs felt strong and powerful, my calves ready for more work.

So I just kept right on running, going one more whole lap plus just a little bit extra for good measure.

Cruising to a stop, I caught my breath and pulled out my cell phone to check the distance on my app. Immediately I texted my sister: *I just ran 3.1 miles! Do you know what that means?*

Her response was almost instantaneous: *You just ran a 5K!*

Two months ago I wasn't a runner. Hell, two months ago I don't even know if I could have run, but here I was running 3.1 miles. Not only running 3.1 miles, but running 3.1 *spontaneous, unplanned* miles.

In that moment, endorphins and pride coursing through my body, it was decided:

I was going to sign up for a race.

3
Hills Like White Elephants

Living in Cleveland not only means I get to call *THE BEST CITY IN THE ENTIRE WORLD* my home, but it also means living in a rich and illustrious city with a history lesson around every corner. Including the story of Jeptha Homer Wade.

Originally from New York, industrialist and philanthropist Jeptha Homer Wade made his money as a telegraph pioneer in the 1850s, overseeing the construction of thousands of lines of communication all across the Midwest. By 1856, after a series of acquisitions and consolidations of smaller companies, these lines morphed into the Western Union Telegraph Company. Wade, the company's first general agent, eventually became president of Western Union in 1866.

Telegraphy was sort of like the nineteenth-century version of texting, in that it was a long-distance, text-based form of communication different from, say, the telephone. Before this, friends and family had to communicate via letters, delivered by hand (or boat, or horse, or some other antiquated mode of transportation that we would scoff at using seriously now). Mail delivery services could take weeks just to go one way, then the same time for a response, and that's if traveling conditions were ideal.

These days, single people are ready to move on if their latest Tinder swipe doesn't respond back within a matter of minutes, so just imagine trying to date that way.

(Then again, I'm a ripe old thirty-five-year-old who is already settled and Tinder intimidates the hell out of me, so dating by letters doesn't sound too shabby after all. If nothing else, if I didn't like the response, or didn't get one, I could just pretend it got lost or something.)

Needless to say, the introduction of a faster transatlantic mode of communication was a Big Deal and ol' Jeptha Homer Wade was in on the ground floor.

Around the same time as Western Union's launch, Wade and his family settled in Cleveland, opting to live in a mansion along the city's famous Euclid Avenue.

Running northeast through the downtown district, the lavish Euclid Avenue was internationally known as the home of distinguished residents during the late nineteenth and into the early twentieth century. The elm-lined street, with its opulent mansions and extravagant gardens, attracted enlightened and illustrious men of the era, including John D. Rockefeller and John Hay, personal secretary to Abraham Lincoln. So posh were its denizens, that it was often compared to Paris's Avenue des Champs-Elysées.

Jeptha Homer Wade was among this avenue's inhabitants and owned a substantial piece of land on the east side of the city. In 1872, sensing an opportunity, he began to convert that land into a public park. Ten years later, he offered seventy-five acres to the city, with the understanding that any further development would keep the land in use as a public park that would always be open to the public.

This gift, along with the small herd of white-tailed American deer that came with it, became the inauspicious beginnings of Cleveland's first zoo.

As the city grew in size and scope, the area surrounding Wade Park branched out, eventually becoming the city's focal point for cultural facilities. This meant that when the Cleveland Museum of Art opened in 1916 and the city wanted to take advantage of the lush green space of Wade Park to enhance the museum's exterior ambiance, the city decided to relocate the zoo from its East Side location to its current location on the West Side.

Today, the zoo's more than 2,000 animals make their home inside the perimeters of a 185-acre park situated on the south West Side of the city. Part of the larger urban metroparks, the zoo is located in a valley visible from the freeways rising high above. Homes along the neighboring streets have open views to peer down into the animal homestead. Full of green grass, walking paths, and a wide variety of animals to view, the Cleveland Metroparks Zoo is a substantial entertainment attraction within the city, garnering over one million visitors a year.

Growing up in the suburbs of Northeast Ohio there was inevitably that one warm day in May towards the end of every school year when my classmates and I all piled into a big, bright yellow school bus and were driven up to the big, bright city for a field trip.

I loved going on field trips as a kid, mostly because it was the one day a year my mom let me pack something other than a boring sandwich for lunch. Field trips meant Lunchables, and whenever I had one coming up my mom took me to the store and let me pick out whatever variety of Lunchables I wanted. I gazed at the neon yellow packaging with stars in my eyes, completely overwhelmed by the sheer number of options available to me under the fluorescent lights of the refrigerated section of the grocery store.

Field trips to the Cleveland Metroparks Zoo felt like an extra special adventure to a young me, reaching almost to the level of an exotic safari, as not only did I get to eat a Lunchables, carefully alternating the unnaturally round slices of processed cheese with the unnaturally round slices of processed meat so they looked like a stack of poker chips on a cracker, but my classmates and I also got to eat at little picnic tables located right next to the animal exhibits. Seeing those magnificent beasts up close and in person, especially the lions opening their wide mouths to yawn in the noonday sun, shaking out their large manes, was a totally different experience than eating lunch at home with my pet cat, Max.

As I was about to enter middle school, the Cleveland Metroparks Zoo opened a new indoor tropical exhibit, aptly called the RainForest. My family planned our first visit for right after opening day.

The RainForest was, and still is, two levels with winding staircases built into faux tree trunks. Making my way up that very first time, I felt like I was in the coolest treehouse ever. It was like something out of *Swiss Family Robinson*. At the center of the building is a large glass-enclosed habitat for the orangutans, who climb high above us into the RainForest's impressive geodesic dome.

Experiencing the RainForest for the first time was nothing short of magical, and the magnetism of the entire menagerie imprinted itself on a young me; even as a thirtysomething woman, I still find the ability to go toe-to-toe with the beasts of the wild to be pretty awesome. I love to watch graceful giraffes stretch their gaits across the green grass of their open paddock, necks held high; or lazy lions luxuriate in the warmth, like a domesticated cat who has found a patch of sunlight in the house; or polar bears dive beneath the crystal clear blue waters of their personal pool.

Even now, far removed from the tiny desks of my kindergarten classroom, living a proper grown-up life where fun field trips are no longer an option, I still love spending an easy summer afternoon at the Cleveland Metroparks Zoo standing among the grand majesty of nature's creatures.

In the summer of 2012, as I was beginning my running journey, I was looking for races in the Cleveland area and saw a listing for the Running with a Mission 5K, which would be held at the Cleveland Metroparks Zoo. As soon as I read the location, I zeroed-in on it as the perfect opportunity for my official racing debut. I mean, hello, I was going to get to run around all those awesome animals. How cool was *that?*

I totally admit now that choosing a race based entirely on the fact that it was the site of hazy, halcyon days of classroom field trips and whimsical bouts of nostalgia sounds sweet and sentimental. Sappy, even. Because as it turns out, nostalgia isn't the smartest way to go about choosing your first race, because while taking a stroll down remembrance road, the mature memory will filter out some of the more prominent geological features of the landscape. Rose-colored glasses will shade the narrative, focusing on the peaks and high points of the journey, ignoring or outright forgetting the valleys.

In this case, my memory completely abandoned all recollection of the not just one, but *two* hills that make up the zoo's loop around the park. Because, that's how a loop works, right?

The course for this race is undeniably scenic. Beginning at the entrance near Monkey Island, the zoo's footpath takes visitors past the African Savannah, which includes zebras and giraffes, and up a short incline to the Northern Trek, a small summit where visitors can see the tigers, bears, and . . . well, the lions are actually down by their African companions, but close enough.

From the Northern Trek, visitors make their own trek past the wolves and down to Waterfowl Lake, which sits at the heart of the park. Anchored on one side of the lake is a Victorian-themed ice cream parlor in a small, Victorian building called Wade Hall. This building was the original barn for the deer that came with the property when Jeptha Wade gave it to the city, making it one of the oldest zoo buildings in North America.

At this point, visitors are left with a choice of how they would like to get up to the top of the big hill which takes them to the Primate, Cat, and Aquatics building. Option one is the small hill tucked back behind the lake in a grove of trees or Option Two, is a large—and long—multilevel deck walk that goes right up to the back of the exhibit.

After circling the building, the path goes down a very large—and long—hill, winding through the Australian Adventure corridor and the African Elephant Crossing before bringing visitors back to the Welcome Plaza near the front entrance. This particular path can be walked, but due to the topographical nature of the park, the zoo utilizes a tram system for visitors who want to save their legs a bit of work.

With the offer of a tram, very few walk up all the hills and even fewer take advantage of an opportunity to *run* up them.

Being a runner means I am constantly learning. After multiple 5Ks, 10Ks, and half marathons, I'm still learning things about this sport. New situations arise, new challenges present themselves, and I have to figure out how best to deal and (hopefully) come out successful on the other side of the finish line.

Every race proves a new opportunity to educate myself about what it means to be a runner and what it means to run. Races in particular provide a steady stream of chances to gain new information and, unsurprisingly, my racing debut came with a very steep learning curve.

The very first hard-learned lesson came swift and quick, leaving me unbalanced, overwhelmed, and unprepared all before I'd even had coffee the morning of the race.

Jill's first running-related lesson: always read course maps very, very carefully.

What I didn't take into account when I signed up for the Running with a Mission 5K is that while that big footpath loop around the park seems long in distance, it's actually not. Like, not at all. Since returning to Cleveland, I'd visited the zoo a handful of times and it's one of those situations when, because I would spend all day walking, my comprehension of the size and scope of the zoo was going to be a bit skewed, making it feel much bigger than it actually is. In reality, that loop is only about one and a half miles around. The RainForest, which felt monstrous when I was little, is not nearly as large as I remember. That staircase carved out of a tree that seemed to rise to the heavens, feels small when I return as an adult. It's more like a novelty staircase on a playground than a set of stairs meant to be utilized by adults as well.

Perhaps unsurprisingly, running the Running with a Mission 5K wasn't my first foray into the area of misplaced nostalgia. Like most kids, my sister and I each had a favorite movie when we were growing up and we would beg our parents to rent that VHS from the video store constantly. As in Every. Single. Weekend. (Yes, I am old enough to remember the VHS and Betamax format war, the precursor of the already outdated DVD and Blu-ray format war.) In the 1980s, little me would kneel in front of the VCR, blonde pigtails high on my head, excited to watch the Strawberry Shortcake movie my mom had rented for me.

On many a family-pizza Friday night, my sister and I wanted to go to the video store in downtown Hudson to rent our favorite movies. My particular favorite was the David Bowie–led masterpiece *Labyrinth*.

I can say that it is without a doubt one of the best children's films to come out of the 1980s, which is saying something as that particular decade was full of really dark, really twisted films aimed at children, and I was obsessed with each and every one. Upon reflection, that probably speaks to my current personality more than any other possible pop culture influence I had growing up.

Right, okay, so there's a movie. In this case, *Labyrinth,* and every Friday night I was begging my parents to go to the video store in town to rent it because I am just *obsessed* and had to see it again and again (and again). And because VHS tapes were only rarely ever "priced to own" at the time, the only option was to rent it from the video store. As I child, I never got to own my own Bowie masterpiece

But kids grow up and film tastes adapt and evolve. The small collection of VHS tapes that went off to college with me soon started to be exchanged for DVDs. As technology also adapted and changed, video stores fell to the wayside and eventually the ability to stream the latest blockbuster from below the pile of blankets and cats on my bed was a reality. I can't even remember the last DVD I bought.

(No, wait. I lied. It was the *Star Wars* trilogy to replace the VHS tapes I bought shortly after the films were remastered and rereleased into theaters back in the early 2000s. And by *Star Wars* trilogy I, of course, mean the original—Episodes IV, V, and VI. Because Fuck Jar Jar Binks.)

Anyway.

A VHS copy of *Labyrinth* was my very first ever Amazon.com purchase, made in late 1999. A few years later I replaced it with a DVD edition, placing it on the shelf at the beginning of the alphabetized-by-title Ls, where it soon sat collecting dust because pushing a single button on my Apple TV to see the latest Netflix offerings was way easier.

But fast-forward to January 10, 2016. After spending an entire day crying and listening to *Space Oddity* on a Spotify loop, I decide the only way to properly honor the late, great David Bowie was to go home and dig out that DVD. I'm grieving the death of a man I never met, surely engaging in some Muppet Magic will cure what ails me.

Only . . . something isn't quite right. As an adult, re-watching this film, the one I was absolutely enamored with as a child, something feels off. As though across the time and space of two decades, some of the magic has dissipated and been lost in translation. For one thing, while Jennifer Connelly would eventually go on to win an Academy Award for her work in 2001's *A Beautiful Mind,* this particular film is maybe not the best example of her acting chops. Then again, her entire supporting cast is made up of a baby, a rock star, and puppets, so I can't really say she had an easy job with this one.

Really though, it's just so *weird.* Way weirder than I remembered.

No wonder my parents hated having to rent it every week and watch it so often.

So, as I'm constantly relearning, perception can be entirely age-related.

≈≈≈

Now back to running: because of the layout of the Cleveland Metroparks Zoo, in order for a 5K to take place and meet that distance, all runners needed to run that loop *twice.* As such, all runners would be forced to run those hills twice. So it wasn't just two hills I had to contend with, it was now four.

Only, I didn't realize that when I signed up. I didn't realize that through any of my weeks and months of runs leading up to the race. In fact, I didn't realize that until the morning of the race, when I was getting ready and checking over all the race details one more time.

And that is when I noticed the small little notation in the bottom corner of the course map uploaded on the website that said runners would have to run the course twice.

Well then.

Now, some race day surprises are not so fun. Like winning a gift card to a local restaurant at a post-race raffle. Or anxiously watching the weather in the days preceding the race only to wake up to absolutely perfect running weather.

Other race day surprises, not so fun. Like finding out I had to tackle a set of hills twice. A set of hills I was woefully unprepared for.

Remember, I hadn't followed any sort of formal training plan for this race. I used Couch to 5K to start running and then, after registering for the race, I just kept running, lacing up and pounding the pavement a couple of times a week.

But that's all it was: running. There was no structure, no set or planned mileage. There certainly wasn't anything more involved than just stepping outside my front door and running around the block a couple of times or doing a couple of laps at nearby Edgewater Park.

Hills were not, and still are not, my forte, but back in 2012, a month before my first race, they weren't even on my radar. Any "hill work" I did was purely accidental: if I decided to run somewhere that just happened to have hills, it was one thing. But actually planning a workout running up and down hills—yeah, no. I didn't even know that was something people actually did.

With all of those runs in May and June, I had been working towards finishing the 5K with a time of 45 minutes, which would require running those 3.1 miles in just under 15 minutes each. Not fast by any stretch of the imagination, but definitely faster than the 16-minute miles I was running in the weeks leading up to race day.

Aside from the hills, a little thing called weather can throw a wrench in the works.

That's right, the bane of many a runner's existence: *humidity*. It was the middle of June after all, and summer was in full swing. I had started running indoors on the treadmill in February. My outdoors runs started in cool and breezy spring, when it's the Goldilocks of weather, neither too hot nor too cold. Of *course* running in the summer would be different. Heat and humidity can affect the body in numerous ways, and while the body can and will adapt and change to its environment as needed, sometimes that environment is just too powerful and will overcome.

Letting this new information regarding weather and pace sink in, I realized a little too late that I was still very much a novice when it came to running. I signed up for the race thinking it was all just a matter of, y'know, *running* and while to some extent it is, there are so many other things I still needed to learn.

Running, it turns out, is a continual learning process as I was reminded, yet again, when I looked at the course map more closely. First lesson learned.

My next experience came from learning what to do on race day.

Going to a new race always makes me a little nervous, even now. Where do I go for packet pick-up? What's the parking and traffic situation going to be like? How much time do I need to give myself? How many other runners are going to be there? I tend to overcompensate in all of those areas, leaving the apartment much earlier than I need to in order to make sure I have plenty of time to get to where I need to go. Usually this is okay because, if nothing else, it gives me plenty of time to hit the restroom before lining up at the start line. Other times, though, it turns into a situation where I am hanging out in my car for a while, because it's the dead of winter, and there is snow on the ground, and the race is being held at a location without an indoor waiting facility.

But for my first race, I had absolutely no idea what to expect. In all fairness, how could I? It's not like I had done this sort of thing before.

I went to bed early the night before, hoping to get a good night's sleep, but nerves made it hard to sleep. In the morning, I was still far too nervous to really eat, but I knew I needed to get something into my body if I wanted to keep it fueled and fit for the run ahead, so I managed to eat a frozen whole-grain waffle with peanut butter and a banana. After getting dressed in black yoga pants and a pink tank top, I got in my car and drove the few miles over to the Cleveland Metroparks Zoo.

The zoo's parking lot is massive, and whenever I go to the zoo as a visitor, I always end up needing to park what feels like miles and miles away. That morning, however, I was able to snag a spot in the front of the lot, right by the zoo's main entrance.

After parking, I got out of my car and followed the crowd towards the small, white tent that had been erected outside the entrance. A woman stood behind a table that was covered with bibs, official-looking large black numbers predominant against the stark white background.

She asked my name and, after checking it against a master list, turned towards some cardboard boxes and from one of them retrieved a white plastic drawstring bag. Inside was a small collection of coupons to local businesses who were sponsors for the race and also a bright blue race shirt. I fingered the soft sleek fabric and knew this was one of the fancy tech shirts that often come at bigger races, but rarely at small races like a local 5K. I put the shirt back in the bag and turned back to the volunteer. She handed me a bib, a set of small safety pins, and a little plastic square-shaped disc that had two holes in the top corners.

Blankly, I stared at the disc, completely flummoxed.

Because I am a librarian, research is kind of my thing, so I spent the weeks leading up to the race looking up information on what to expect with my first race. Things like what to eat (and what not to eat), what to wear (and what not to wear), where to line up, etcetera. The bib was easy and the most obvious part: it gets pinned somewhere on the front so I can be quickly and easily identified by my number, and it's important to pin it in all four corners to keep it stationary. But this disc was new and hadn't come up in any of my research.

After a few seconds of silent uneducated guesswork, I finally looked up at the volunteer. She met my eyes.

"It's your timing chip," she patiently explained. "It goes on your shoe. The holes are for your laces."

Oh. Right. My *timing chip*. That magical device that will alert those that need to know when I cross the start line and then the finish line. This is the first time I would ever learn my speed and ability from a verified source and not just some free app on my phone which may or may not be accurate.

The other data point I'd be learning that day was how I stacked up against other runners.

Not that it was a huge deal or anything: for me, running is a solo sport. Since that moment I took that first step at a speed faster than walking, I had found my happy place. The cliché about running being cheaper than therapy turned out to be true.

But I was still curious to know how I'd fare against other runners.

Since this was not just my first race but my first time running with other runners, I didn't know what my performance would be like in the grand scheme of things. I knew I was slower than most runners and it was unlikely that I'd manage to squeak out ahead of the other Female Runners age thirty to thirty-five to place in my age group, but I didn't think my pace was anything to be concerned about.

I stepped away from the tent, letting the runners behind me move forward to get their own packets. There was a row of park benches sitting against the wall of the building. I propped my right foot up on one of them and undid the laces of my shoe and slid the timing chip onto them, then retied my laces. Damn, I felt legit. Timing chip in place, I took the short walk back to my car to drop the rest of my packet off, then headed into the zoo.

From all that research I knew that because of my slower speed race etiquette dictates I should line up near the back of the pack, so as to not get in the way of those faster runners in the front. We stood near Monkey Island and while waiting for the race to officially start, I watched the black-and-white Colobus Monkeys jump and shriek around their habitat, sharing in the excitement for the day.

Then, after what felt like forever, the gun went off and we started running. Almost immediately, the majority of the other runners surged far, far ahead of me, but I didn't really think anything of it. All I was thinking about was the fact that I was *running*. In a *race*. With a bib and a timing device and a finish line and everything. This was legit.

Passing by the Rhinoceros Building, I heard joyful shouts and looked up to my left where high above, the front of the pack was already making their way up the first hill, led by a man clearly in a familiar position. With a quick glance over my shoulder I breathed an internal sigh of relief when I saw a couple of people straggling behind me.

Whew. Wasn't in last place.

The path before me started its incline up towards the Northern Trek and the change in topography slowed me down slightly, but I kept moving forward. I followed the course up and around the wolves, then down towards Waterfowl Lake. Passing Wade Hall, I suddenly had a not-small hankering for ice cream. The race had started promptly at 9 a.m. and the summer sun was out high in the cloudless sky. Yet, here I was, running in the heat.

Yeah, ice cream was starting to sound *really* good right about now.

Shortly past Waterfowl Lake was the Koala Building and, a bit beyond that, the turn that would take me up the hill towards the Primate, Cat, and Aquatics buildings.

As I crested the hill and continued running towards the building, I spotted a water station ahead which was a welcome relief, because it was June, it was the height of summer, and it was hot outside and I was *running* for fuck's sake, so, yes, water, please. *GIVE ME ALL THE WATER.*

Here was another learning opportunity because, as it turns out, attempting to run and drink water at the same time doesn't work out too well. It's a lot harder than it looks.

Being parched and tired, I grabbed one of those paper cups from a volunteer and, without stopping, took a huge gulp. I then spent the next ten or so seconds choking and then another ten seconds trying to catch my breath again.

I was mortified beyond belief and glanced at the other runners around me, wondering if anyone happened to see me make a fool of myself while trying to stay hydrated. They all were in the zone and completely ignoring me, but I still felt like a total idiot.

I followed the path around the Primate, Cat, and Aquatics buildings, knowing the big hill was ahead of me. Luckily I only had to run down it, not up. But it's a steep hill, the kind of steep where it's tricky to regain much, if any, of the speed lost from going up previous hills because all focus was on not tripping over my feet and falling down the hill.

With the double loop of the course, at the end of the hill there were signs directing all of the participants. Along with the 5K run there was also a 1.5 mile walking event which only required one pass at the loop. At the bottom of the hill, the walkers and the 5K runners finishing their second loop were directed towards the finish line while those of us who were just starting our second loop were directed back towards the front entrance to run the route again.

Stationed in front of the entrance, just past the finish line, were all of the volunteers and spectators. It was a huge, very loud group at that: as I ran past them they cheered and hollered encouragement, cowbells ringing spiritedly. This was the halfway point of my very first 5K and their support rang in my ears, pushing me forward to tackle those hills all over again.

A huge, stupid, toothy grin spread across my face and I was so glad I was wearing sunglasses because I felt myself start to well up with a mix of emotions.

By this point, my legs were starting to get really tired and not just from the running: the mistake of not reading the course map carefully enough was starting to catch up with me as the reality of my situation began to sink in.

My exhausted legs managed to make it up the first incline without too much extra effort, but by the time I got up and around the Northern Trek exhibit and back down to Waterfowl Lake, I knew there was no way in hell I was going to be able to run up that second hill for a second time. Knowing the water station was at the top might have been enough to motivate me mentally, but my body was just not physically able to do it.

Feeling a bit defeated, I had to do the thing I didn't want to do: I walked up the hill.

Pumping my arms at my side, I power-walked that hill as much as I could but I was hot and I was tired and my poor legs were doing far more work than they were prepared to do.

Coming down the big hill for that final push of distance, I was greeted by several other runners who had already finished and were now walking around the zoo since our registration included admission for the day. As I passed by them on my way to the finish line they called out words of encouragement and support, telling me I was almost done and to just keep going.

Following the path as it curved around the kangaroo exhibit, I spotted the inflatable arch parked near the entrance. Knowing how close I was to finishing, literally able to see that final stop up ahead, I dug down deep and picked up my pace as much as I could. Granted, I was running downhill so gravity did most of the work, but whatever.

With the crowd of spectators cheering, I crossed that finish line with a roar in my ears. Six months ago I considered running something out of reach and here I was, finishing my first ever 5K race.

After passing over the finish line, I paused for a minute to catch my breath, standing still just long enough to let my legs rest. When I started to make my way towards the pavilion where the post-race snacks and water were, I saw a familiar face standing near the finish line.

Waiting at the end was my college roommate Megan, who was not only a runner, but a runner who happened to work for the company sponsoring the race. She had finished long before I did, but knowing I was running and knowing that this was my first race, she had stayed around and hovered near the finish line to be there when I was done.

Referencing the course and hills, she exclaimed, "You picked a beast for your first one!"

Laughing, and very grateful it was all over, I nodded and told her I did, yes, though it was completely unintentional.

We walked to the pavilion together where I got my banana, sat at one of the picnic tables, and started calling my parents and sister to let them all know I was done. They all asked me what my time was and I honestly couldn't tell them: I had completely forgotten I was being timed and hadn't even really paid attention to the clock posted near the finish line. I had some vague recollection that I finished somewhere in the 47-minute vicinity.

Megan headed out soon after and I walked around the zoo for a bit, although my legs were far too tired for a long day of walking so I soon headed home.

The rest of the weekend was a blur, as I was still riding high on the adrenaline and pride of my accomplishment. By the time I got to work on Monday, race results hadn't been posted yet and I spent all morning hitting the refresh button on my computer, anxious to see how I had fared.

Finally, the race results page changed and a link appeared. Taking a deep breath I clicked the new link open and started scrolling down the page, looking for my name.

When I arrived at the zoo that morning, I had hoped to finish in 45 minutes. Had I been better prepared for those hills (or, y'know, picked a flatter course), I probably could have achieved that goal. My first 5K took me 47:40 to finish, which came out to an average mile pace of 15:23.

Considering I'd been running 16-minute miles in the days prior to the race and considering those hills and the heat, I was perfectly pleased with my time. Then, looking at the rest of the list I saw something I hadn't noticed before: out of 362 people who crossed the start, I was the 362nd person to cross the finish line.

Yup: I had come in last place at my first race.

Life really is nothing more than a series of decisions that parade before us over the course of time. The shape our life takes depends on the choices we make, the paths we take each moment of every day.

45

Some decisions, some choices, seem far more momentous than others: Where do I live? What career path do I follow? Who do I marry?

Other decisions, other choices, are more innocuous, but it is often these decisions that have a greater impact in guiding our journey because it's these simple decisions that compound as we make them every single second of every single moment of every single day. It is not the Friday nights or Saturday evenings that determine who we are and where we go: it is the Thursday afternoons or Monday mornings that mentor and counsel our being into a full-fledged sense of self.

When I knew that I had to change my lifestyle, it followed that I had a decision to make, one that at the time didn't seem like a big deal. I mean, I'd given this whole running experiment a good ol' college try, right? I'd done the treadmill running, I'd done the outside in the park running, I'd even signed up for and finished an honest-to-goodness, real live race.

And I'd come in last place.

What are the odds of that happening at a runner's first race? I mean, really. Over 350 people were there and I was *the very last person* to finish.

When I posted my time on social media, some of my more experienced runner friends said that with that time and place I had clearly been running with some serious runners because they had all run races where that time was still in the back of the pack, but definitely not last place.

I had no way of knowing it at the time, but that 15:23 mile average would not be my slowest time as a runner. Since then, I've run many a 5K, 10K, and three half marathons and some of those races have, for various reasons and circumstances, been finished with slower paces. In some cases, significantly slower paces.

But I didn't know that. All I had to go on was the current data I had before me, which was that I was a slow runner who came in last place.

Of course, that's the nature of races, right? Someone comes in first place and someone comes in last place. That's just how these things work. Someone comes in first place and someone comes in last place and at this particular race on this particular day, I was in last place. Of the 362 people who showed up at the Cleveland Metroparks Zoo on that day, 361 people crossed that finish line before me.

But—and here's the big but—*what about all those people who didn't even cross the start line to begin with?*

Life is a series of moments and decisions and in that moment, I decided that finishing last trumped all other scenarios, including not even starting.

So I came in last place. So what? Was I really going to let one race mark my entire running career? Was I really going to let those 361 other people who beat me on the course beat me again by dropping out of running altogether? That would be silly, right? Not just silly, but kind of dumb considering how much I'd spent on those fancy running shoes a couple of months ago.

I mean, if nothing else, I had to run at least one more race to make sure this race and this last place finish wasn't the only mark on my entire running record.

But only after checking the course map first.

4
Homecoming

About a month after my last-place finish in the race at the zoo, I ran another 5K, this time in nearby Strongsville, Ohio. The Race for Wellness 5K was put on by the Cleveland Clinic, one of two major hospital systems within the city. I picked it mostly for location, Strongsville being not too far from my apartment. In a busy summer, that particular race weekend fit easily into my schedule.

Ironically, despite most assuredly reading the course map before signing up, I was still confronted on race day with a monstrous hill. It was a simple out-and-back course and the halfway mark moved swiftly up a giant incline, then came right back down just as quickly. My parents were able to attend this race and at the finish line, my mom, having heard about the hills at the zoo, told me she overheard other runners talk about being surprised at the hill, so at least it wasn't just me this time.

The rest of the Race for Wellness 5K course was flat and I don't know if it was because of that or I had just gotten naturally faster, but I managed to shave almost a whole minute off of my mile time, making for a nearly three-minute faster 5K time.

With two 5Ks completed, I was beginning to get the hang of this whole racing thing and finally really starting to feel like a real runner.

It was summer, with the sun rising early in the morning and setting late at night, leaving plenty of time in my schedule for running before work in the mornings and after dinner on the weekends.

Running was no longer something I was just trying on. Now, running was something I was doing whenever and wherever I could. I found myself setting my alarm clock earlier and earlier each morning to get runs in before work and sleeping in on the weekends was starting to lose its appeal. I'd rather take advantage of the day and the sun and the nearby parks and run my little heart out. To put this in perspective: BR (Before Running) Jill spent her summer weekends hiding her pale skin from the sun, cycling through her latest Netflix obsession. AR (After Running) Jill was now working out *and* working on her tan (well, no, I was working on my burn because despite now being active and outside more, I can't magically gift myself new skin). In other words, running was becoming second nature to me, like walking or breathing or showing off my vast archive of random film trivia.

(Seriously, it's amazing I manage to fit anything else into my memory at this point.)

Between the endorphins and the swag associated with the sport, I was also starting to become a little addicted to the excitement of race day. At that point I had run my first race in June and my second in July, and it was while looking through lists of upcoming August races in the area that I stumbled upon one that caught my eye in an unexpected way. It should have been an obvious find but I still caught my breath when I realized what it would mean. Reading the description and location details more, I knew this was the one. As in The One. Turn on the neon red sign and flash that baby over Broadway, The One. Twelve years and two 5Ks later, it was finally time to tackle the finish line that had eluded me since I was a teenager.

Right, so, to better understand the importance of this particular race, I need to share some necessary background information related to both the city that raised me and my place there.

(Spoiler alert: I didn't really fit in.)

Besides the infamous running of the Annual Mile each year, the closest I ever came to the track at my school was each Friday night during football season. But I wasn't there to cheer on the football team from the stands, sporting the district colors of blue and white. No, I was there as a member of the marching band. Because, of course I was. I started playing the flute in fifth grade, slowly progressing through middle school and high school bands. I was never the best of my section; I fit comfortably within the middle of the ranks and perfectly content with that place, mostly because I was too lazy to do the work required to advance my position. While my peers spent their free time practicing the required music, I'd spend my free time, well usually not playing my flute at all, but if I did, I was usually playing simplified flute versions of Disney songs and Broadway musicals. Given my established aversion to athletics, marching band wasn't my first choice of extracurriculars but spending the fall semester at football games was the only way a band student was allowed to spend the spring semester sitting on stage for concert band. So every weekend in autumn, I dressed in my heavy white polyester uniform and marched across football fields across Northeast Ohio during halftime.

Let me be clear about the fact that I never paid attention to the actual football game happening in front of me. My freshman year Hudson had a really good football team, although I only know that because the marching band season extended into November when we had to literally freeze our asses off on snow-covered fields for the play-offs. I'm not kidding about the freezing part, either: because of the nature of our instruments, many of the woodwind sections–flutes included–had to cut the tips off of our very thin gloves. This meant exposing our fingers to a metal instrument while outdoors. In winter. In Ohio. This did not endear me to the sport.

Our halftime show was the only time I was ever paying attention to the events on the field—the rest of the game, my girlfriends and I would sing show tunes, slowly (and loudly) working our way through the entire catalogs of Stephen Sondheim, Andrew Lloyd Webber, and Stephen Schwartz. Because, I mean, really. What else were we going to do? Actually watch the game? Please.

Despite attending every single varsity game between freshman and senior year of high school, it took well into my thirties before I actually learned the rules of football.

Some people letter in sports. I lettered in theater and band and I would have lettered in choir if I had started it earlier.

Oh yeah. I was *that* kid in high school.

To be fair, I came from an educational environment that strongly supported the arts and academics. Our quarterback went to an Ivy League school and most people came to the stadium each Friday night *because* of the band, not in spite of it. One of my classmates got a perfect 1600 on the SAT (before it was graded out of 2400) and the school recognized his achievement at one of our regular pep rallies.

Still, walking the halls of Hudson High School I often felt like a stranger in a strange land. My study halls were for reading books I had checked out from the public library (where I also worked) and writing fan fiction with friends based on our favorite sci-fi television shows (we put Mulder and Scully together long before Chris Carter got around to it). At lunch, we had a big set of tables off to the side of the main eating area in the cafeteria. We may have been considered the outcasts and misfits, but we certainly outnumbered some of the other cliques in our school. Funny how that works out sometimes.

But for all the things that separated me from my peer group growing up, there was one thing that brought us all together. Something that crossed socioeconomic backgrounds, grade point averages, and extra-curricular activities: a strong desire to leave our hometown.

It must be a Northeast Ohio thing 'cause, I mean, look at LeBron James. Granted, he took a more . . . dramatic exit than most, leaving in flames (quite literally, with fumes from burning jerseys following him all the way to Miami). But, y'know, he just had some shit he had to work out. Like most twentysomethings. As adolescents, we think we know everything, we think we know better, and we think we'll find greener grass on the other side of the Ohio borders. At sixteen, my main motivator in life was to get out of Ohio, although I would have settled for just getting out of Hudson, which I did when I went away to college.

After receiving my BFA in creative writing from Bowling Green State University, I returned to Hudson and once again made it my goal to get out of Ohio. This time I was successful and moved to Kentucky for a period of time that included graduate school.

See, I'm kind of like LeBron. I moved south, played in the

grown-up leagues for a while, then graduated and after graduating, I looked around and realized something was missing. I made my pilgrimage back to Northeast Ohio, only this time settling in the big city of Cleveland, and I quickly made a life for myself that includes occasional visits to my hometown, where my parents still live.

I was raised in upper middle class white suburbia, although I grew up on the South Side of town, not on the North where all of the ritzy McMansions can be found. It's a city steeped in a rich history, dating back to its 1799 founding. Imagine, if you will, that some eighteenth century wizard figured out how to take a quaint, picturesque New England hamlet and just lift the entire thing and plop it down in the northeast corner of Ohio. Because that's pretty much what happened, minus the whole wizard part. Driving through Hudson is like driving through a Norman Rockwell painting.

When I was in high school, while there was small track in the backfields where we ran the mile every year, the school did not have a proper football stadium. But in 2009, the city decided it was time the varsity football team had a proper football stadium on the school's property. Three years later, the city broke ground on the $5.5 million project, which was completely funded by the community and private donations. The stadium was ready and open to the public just a few months later in August 2012, just in time for football season. The large complex includes all-weather turf with seating for 5,000 and a track.

This was a momentous occasion for Hudson, and to celebrate the grand opening of the brand-new stadium, several events were scheduled across the city, one of which was a 5K.

The Veteran's Memorial 5K, my third race, weighed more heavily on me than the previous two combined because the race both began and ended inside the stadium. That meant that this alumni, the one who used to walk the mile every year, was going to be *running* on the new high school track.

In the weeks leading up to the race I was balancing carefully between excitement and anxiety, all while still trying to contend with running in the heat.

As a runner, it's so natural to want to let pace be a defining data point. It's quantifiable, like a number on a scale. It's something that can be tracked and examined over time. When it comes to running, there are very few things that can be monitored in that same manner. Therefore, speed is what comparatively defines runners.

So what does it mean for a runner who is already slow that external forces, like heat and humidity, are slowing her down even more? I can't control the weather (sadly) and I certainly can't control the temperature, but both of these things were causing me to not run at what I would consider my best.

Before the Running with a Mission 5K back in June, I let this get under my skin. I let myself, and my identity as a runner, be defined by a set of numbers. A "good" pace left me feeling elated, while a "bad" pace left me feeling like a failure.

It all was arbitrary, of course. *Good* and *bad* don't have any real set definition and one runner's "bad" run is another runner's "good." This can be especially true as a back-of-the-pack runner when confronted with other runners complaining about running a 12- or 13-minute mile and thinking *I'd trade all of my finisher's medals to run that.*

(Okay, well, I wouldn't *really* trade away all of my finisher's medals, but you get the point.)

But since it's arbitrary, that also means it's all subjective. So, yes, a faster runner's bad pace is my good pace (and, vice versa, my bad pace is someone else's no good, horrible, very rotten bad pace). We are all running our own races with our own goals and finish lines, whether that's the finish line on the ground or one created in our mind.

Which is why, in the weeks leading up to the Veteran's Memorial 5K, I just stopped worrying about my pace.

Unless a runner is qualifying for the Boston Marathon and chasing that BQT (Boston Qualifying Time, for you running nubes), in the big old grand scheme of things, speed and pace has no real meaning. Oh sure, it was a good idea for me to have goals, and there was nothing wrong if one of those goals was simply to be faster than my last race, but I decided that I no longer was going to let that finish time determine my sense of self or worth as a runner.

Especially not in summer when I can only put so much effort into it before forces way beyond my control have their way with me. All the training and planning in the world can't save a runner when Mother Nature decides to exert some of her power, reminding us all who is *really* in control on race day.

Nope, when it came to racing I was just going to run, and let the timing chips fall where they may.

Granted, I was a brand-new runner and a slow one at that, so it's entirely possible I had no idea what the hell I was talking about. But I was also a runner who fully embraced last place at her first race so I also like to believe I'm runner-wise beyond my years.

The Veteran's Memorial 5K was an early Saturday morning race at the end of August 2012. Since my parents still live in my hometown, I drove to their house the Friday before and spent the night there. The next day I was up early, as was my mom, who has always been an early riser.

Over the past few months I had gotten into a bit of a routine when it came to my pre-race fueling, so I had come to my parents' house prepared with some hard-boiled eggs, yogurt, and a small bagel. Even though I knew there was a chance I'd be able to find most of the same food in my parents' house, I didn't want to take that risk of needing to eat something new right before this race. I was already feeling ridiculously nervous about this race, no need to add more stress by changing up my dietary habits. Runners have a lot of . . . not superstitions per se, but routines and quirks that come out around race day, and food is always a big one. From what we eat the night before to the fuel we use during a race and, yes, even the meal right before a run. Much of it, for me at least, is trial and error. But once an optimal food has been found, even if it's all psychological, it's difficult to break a runner from that habit, hence the need to bring my own breakfast.

With plenty of time to spare, I changed into my running clothes, kissed my mom goodbye, and headed to the high school. My dad was still asleep, but I knew they'd eventually be meeting me at the school.

I parked my car in the lot designated for seniors during the school year and walked over to the new stadium. It was massive, far more state-of-the-art than the stadium I used to play my flute in fifteen years before. The high school, and thus the stadium, is in the middle of a residential area of town and surrounded by a lot of woods. This is the suburbs of Ohio, so there is not much else out there and certainly not any buildings higher than two stories. Light pollution is very limited and the nearby woods create a dense field of darkness all around. This means that when the team is playing at home, those stadium lights can be seen for miles, like a collection of brightly burning suns blazing high above the school.

(The team is talented and has made it to the state play-offs several seasons in a row. We're good, but Ohio isn't exactly Texas country. You wouldn't know that, though, driving towards that stadium on game night. It's like *Friday Night Lights* out there, which I'm pretty sure is exactly the same thing I said the first time I attended a game at the varsity team's new home.)

After picking up my packet, I pinned my bib to my shirt and found a spot along the track fence and just stood there, taking in the atmosphere and magnitude of the new stadium. I get that for most people, even maybe most runners, this didn't seem like that big of a deal. It's not like this was my first race nor was it a big-name race in a fancy destination location. I hadn't spent weeks training, and I wasn't tackling a new distance. This was just some little 5K in some little town in Ohio.

But it was *my* little town. A little town I had spent most of my childhood and a good chunk of my adult life running away from. Here, today, I was still running, but this time I was running in a completely different context and for a completely different reason. I wasn't running away from Hudson or away from the miserable mile from my past; I was running towards my bright and bold future as a runner. I was carving a new path, a new set of miles. I was a new Jill. It was redemption time, baby.

As I waited for my parents to arrive, I leaned against the fence that ran the perimeter of the football field. Other runners were starting to arrive, clustering into small groups on and off the field. I surveyed the wandering crowd, looking for any familiar faces. Not that I really anticipated knowing anyone, but there was always that chance in a small town. Music pumped into my ears from my iPod.

As any harrier will tell you, music for a runner is a very personal choice. Some run with it, some without. I find I have to run with music and I keep a carefully curated collection of songs available for when I workout. As I stood there, gazing up at the bright blue sky, the familiar opening beats of Black Sabbath's "Iron Man" came on and I grinned. As a teenager, the only thing resembling any sort of athletic endeavor I voluntarily put myself through was marching band. Black Sabbath's iconic rock song was the opening number to the first show my freshman classmates and I ever did on that field, a performance we recreated as upperclassmen four years later for the annual Senior Show. Having that song, of all songs, come across the wires, pulled from the depths of thousands of musical options, seemed like a sign from Hermes, the Greek god of Running—I was about to rock (and roll) the hell out of this race.

The course started on the new track, at the heart of the Veteran's Memorial Stadium. While I was waiting for the race to start, a small crowd of spectators had gathered in the stands, my parents included. The stadium stands were so brand-new, the metallic material was blinding as the August sun bounced off them.

When there were only a few minutes left until the start of the race, we all started to find our places on the track. It wasn't a very big race, with just a few dozen runners, but a healthy mix of adults as well as middle school– and high school–aged kids as well. With the high school as the backdrop to the waiting runners, I found my way to the back of the small crowd.

The gun went off and the spectators in the stands started to loudly cheer us on as we all picked up our feet and started towards the back end of the stadium. The course began with a few yards on the track before exiting out the back end of the perimeter fence to a small trail located behind the high school. A trail I hadn't seen or thought about in over ten years but still, a trail I knew I had been on before as it was part of the conditioning running course our gym teachers would take us on in the days leading up to the Annual Mile. Less than a quarter of a mile in and already, nostalgia was taking hold.

The trail took me away from the school, along the far boundary of the high school's campus. Here, I ran against the large expansive green grass at the back end of the school, the baseball and soccer fields to my right. At the end of the trail, the course turned out onto Hudson-Aurora Road, one of the major streets in the community.

Next, after passing beneath the Ohio Turnpike overpass, I ran along the sidewalks of the bustling Hudson-Aurora Road. After a quarter of a mile or so, the course turned left onto the Turnpike Trail for the next mile and a half of the race.

Up until this point, all of my miles had been logged within the confines of a major metropolitan area. These were city miles. Even my beloved Edgewater Park is all open air. Here I was in a dense forest, lush and just so very *green*. So many shades flitted within the peripherals of my vision, the sun cutting bright rays through the available gaps in the canopy high above. Trail running was new to me, (although this really was more of a paved walkway in the middle of a narrow strip of land, heavily populated with tall trees). Because of the trees, I had to be a little more aware of my footing and keep my eyes on the ground for fear that I'd trip over a branch and break my ankle (something that would be quite par for the course given my clumsy sprains), but other than that I felt oddly liberated. Somehow, being enclosed by the trees added an element of freedom I hadn't anticipated. And it was just so *quiet*. No noisy cars from the streets or people all around. The only thing I heard was the natural rustle of leaves in the light breeze and critters who lived there.

After a mile and a half, Turnpike Trail dead-ends into Stow Road and the course turned to the right to run a few yards along it. By this point in the race the crowd had thinned out enough that I hadn't seen another runner ahead or behind me for what felt like hours (although, in reality it was closer to maybe twenty minutes). But I really wasn't worried; the scenery was distracting in its idyllic-ness. The trees were just so green, and I had never before paid much attention to the variety of verdigris that exists. Running alone along the Bicentennial Trail, it felt like I had my own private forest. I knew I had already passed the halfway mark for the 5K, meaning I was already halfway home. I was halfway to conquering the past and overcoming my own fears and insecurities.

As I made my way through the tunnel of trees, I felt the first wave of emotions start to rise up as I considered what I was doing. What I was about to do, in less than a mile and a half.

It wasn't even just the running. Not really. The fact that I was running was more like a small cog in an otherwise bigger machine that had been set in motion decades before. At seventeen, I thought I knew what I wanted out of life and had a pretty certain notion of where I would be by the time I reached my thirties.

Such, of course, is the hubris of youth because nowhere in my life plan was the concept of spending a beautiful Saturday morning at the end of August running a race in my hometown.

But here I was, race bib pinned to the front of my tank top, laces of my shoes tied tight. Feet moving . . . well, maybe not swiftly, but certainly moving as fast as I could get them to go.

I sometimes wonder what teenage me would think of the adult me. If she knew what lies ahead, would she make the same choices as I did, blind to the future? Or, would she take advantage of this certain knowledge and make different, perhaps better, choices? If I had known, as a teenager, that one day I would be a runner, would I have used my years in high school and college to cultivate my love for running at an early age?

Who would I be now if I had discovered this sport earlier in my life? Where would I be, how many miles would I have logged, had I embraced the Annual Mile instead of rebelling against it? My friend and former roommate Megan has run multiple marathons. All those years living with her and I never took advantage of that athleticism, still scarred by too many humiliating physical education classes. Would *I* have multiple marathons under my legs by now? Would those legs be faster than the ones I have right now? (*Probably*, but I also probably wouldn't be writing this memoir either.)

There's always a trade-off. While that certain knowledge would absolutely have some undisputed benefits, small choices like that which seem unimportant have consequences over the narrative arc of a person's life. It's the Butterfly Effect, as every '90s kid learned from Jeff Goldblum in *Jurassic Park*: "A butterfly flaps his wings in Peking and in Central Park you get rain instead of sunshine." Small changes have far-reaching effects.

Had I started running far earlier than I did, my relationship to the sport wouldn't be the only thing different in my life now . . . My aversion to athletics had affected other areas of my life—my relationship with my parents, with my sister, with food and, in turn, my relationship with my body. By not exercising on a regular basis, I spent much of my life struggling with my weight. Job prospects, relationship prospects, it all ties in. It's all a part of the person I am today.

Maybe it's silly to think of these things in such a Big Picture way— as if I have some strange notion that if I had listened to my gym teachers and actually tried to run the mile as early as sixth or seventh grade that now, twenty some years later, I'd be a fucking Boston Qualifier, or some bullshit. Or that Olympic medal winner Shalane Flanagan and I would be BFFs, sharing long runs together on the weekends. But it's an easy fantasy to fall into, especially when I'm full of self-doubt and feeling down on myself because of my speed.

But then I think about the parts of my life I'd be giving up if such a parallel life had come to fruition. There are moments in my history I would not like to relive, but am I willing to accept them when it's *those* moments that shape who I am now?

I often say I'm a constant work in progress, never settling or defining myself. I'm always changing, perpetually challenging myself to be better. I'm a patchwork sewn together with snatches of brief moments over three decades of this thing we call Life. Looking it all over, it's those scary parts, the dark and twisty parts that shine the brightest.

It's those scary, dark, and twisty parts that prompted me to take up running initially. Because it's not sunshine and roses that gets a person weighing over 300 pounds. In my case, it was a lot of misplaced shame and low self-esteem that was dealt with in the form of late-night candy bars and almost daily trips to the drive-through of local fast food restaurants.

If I had never gotten myself in a position where I weighed 311 pounds, my sister would have never written me that email in December of 2010. If she had never written me that email, I never would have set out to lose weight, and if I had never been determined to get to a smaller size, I never would have turned to running as a form of exercise. While it may have taken me a rather circuitous route to get there, but I'd rather have arrived a little late to the party if it meant I could spend my later years there, than have been a guest back in the day who went home before the event really got started.

Because, really, even if I had done well as a runner when I was younger, there's nothing to guarantee that I would have continued as I got older. I could have run the mile in middle and high school, swiftly moving my way around the track in my polyester blue uniform. Maybe I would have even run track and in college gone on to tackle longer distances like Megan, racking up half marathon after half marathon.

Or, maybe, kind of like with my flute playing and the marching band, I would have quit once I was no longer being graded for my participation. Even if I was a natural at it, I don't know if I would have had the motivation and determination at that age to follow it through.

If these were my options—be a faster runner as a teenager who fizzled out before reaching adulthood versus being someone who discovered her love for the activity later on, knowing she had the rest of her life to run, even if at a slower pace . . . I would take the latter option every day of the week. Really, it's not even a question that needs to be asked.

So it was, while running through a forest just a hair's breadth away from my old stomping ground, that I really started to see the forest for the trees.

Glen Echo: a typical quiet, suburban street lined with quaint homes full of families still asleep on this summer morning. It was here that the Bicentennial Trail ended and the final leg of the 5K began. Immediately adjacent to the high school campus, I knew I was closing in on that finish line. I followed the curve of the road until I found myself back on Hudson-Aurora Road. At the intersection I turned right, putting myself back on the long stretch of road outside the high school.

As I neared the mouth of the driveway I looked to the right, towards the school and stadium. Tall pillars of steel rose high against the horizon. The stadium, the finish line, the *track of my high school*, was so close I could practically feel the black rubber beneath my shoes already.

Behind the dark shade of my sunglasses, my eyes started to water.

When I reached the driveway entrance to the high school, I turned right and headed up the slight incline towards the stadium looming in the back of the property. I ran through the adjacent parking lot and through the entrance to the field's fence.

Situated a few yards ahead of me, on the track, was the blue inflatable tunnel used by the varsity football team during home games. When we started, the tunnel had been pushed back into a corner of the fence and I didn't think anything of it. When I looked through the opening I spied the finish line clock, the digital seconds counting up. Clearly, I was meant to run through the tunnel.

This was it. *This was the moment.* There was literally a light at the end of the tunnel. On the other side of that tunnel wasn't just the finish line and hugs from my parents. Running through that tunnel, passing under the front arch with the words HUDSON EXPLORERS emblazoned in big white letters, solidified just how far I had come. From the girl who had walked one mile on the track to the woman who had just run three of them.

I took a deep breath. I took all that teenage angst and low self-esteem and turned it inside out, transforming the negative energy into something positive. Flying through that tunnel I fell down the rabbit hole into my own personal Wonderland.

In 1940, Thomas Wolfe published the novel *You Can't Go Home Again.* In the decades since, his title has entered the American lexicon to signify an antithesis to nostalgia and sentimentality. Youthful wistfulness will never be as Technicolor-esque in our memories as it was in the moment we lived it, but that's not always a bad thing. Sometimes memories too painful to relive seem to burn brighter and we yearn for an opportunity to snuff the flame.

At the same time, who wouldn't love an opportunity to return to the scene of the crime and tell that Bitchy McBitcherson to shut the fuck up when she starts talking smack? Or ask out that one cute guy who was always so nice to you and would chat with you by your locker, but you were always convinced he was just being polite and it took about ten years of life and dating to realize he was so totally flirting with you.

Of course, unless you're a thousand-year-old Gallifrayen who goes by the name "The Doctor" and you tool around time and space in a specially outfitted blue police box, chances are that time travel is a little outside of your areas of expertise. (Then again, if you *are* a thousand-year-old Gallifrayen who goes by the name . . . well, yeah, all of that, um, you should call me.)

All we can, all any of us can do, is keep moving forward and attempt to not let the scars of the past interfere with the future we create for ourselves on a daily basis.

So, yes, I understand Thomas Wolfe's sentiment. But only to an extent. While I support the notion that the memories I have in my mind are shaded with a lens that adds a soft light, I also think it's okay if my remembrance of events past are a little out of focus, a little dull compared to reality. So, sure, I can't relive the past in any meaningful way. I don't have a time machine, be it a DeLorean, a Blue Police Box, or any other untraditional means of time teleportation transportation. I don't have the option of walking the same sidewalks, driving down the same street—too much time has passed at this point.

But that's okay, because those memories, as watered down as they may be, can still be a strong motivator to make changes that set us down a new course. So, with respect to Mr. Wolfe, I have to disagree because I think you can go home again.

And sometimes, if you're only very, very lucky, you even get to run there.

5
Twenty Seconds of Insane Courage

The Veteran's Memorial 5K was only one of several citywide events held in honor of the new varsity stadium. The night before the race, the football team hosted the season opener. And with the start of the new school year, one thing was certain:

Autumn was officially here.

Now anyone who lives outside the sunnier meccas of the US knows all too well that seasonal depression is real, and it affects everyone differently. Even the *seasonal* part of seasonal depression fluctuates from person to person. If asked, most people probably only think of it as a winter affliction since that is when it's most prevalent, but spring and summer seasonal depression exists, even if more rare.

For me, seasonal depression strikes in the fall—sometimes in September, often in October, never in November. By the time my birthday rolls around in mid-November, I have usually managed to maneuver out from under the cloud that keeps my brain foggy and motivation nonexistent.

During this time of my autumnal ennui (or, really, any other time depression decides to strike), just the thought of even thinking about going out for a run requires so much energy that all I want to do is take a nap. That first autumn after I started running was particularly challenging because I knew that I should run, and some part of me even *wanted* to, and I also knew that exercise and endorphins would no doubt be beneficial, but there was just no way I could fight my way out of the harvest haze.

In the past, it had never really mattered if I gave into seasonal ennui because I didn't have any sort of activity or schedule to keep up with. If I wanted to spend an entire weekend immobile in bed going through my entire Netflix queue, I could do so without any sort of repercussions on my training or fitness level.

Granted, that's also the sort of behavior that put me in a position where I once weighed over 300 pounds, but, *tomayto, tomahto.*

Add to this, along with the depression I also have some mild anxiety. This combination doesn't really bode well for my overall sense of self.

The struggle is real.

But as a runner, I have to be thoughtful and aware of how my taking a week or two off is going to have an effect on my running. Things like losing my base become very real concerns. When it comes to starting a new training regiment, nobody wants to start over from scratch.

Now I know the importance of keeping up on mileage, even without an event on the horizon, but back in 2012 I had no idea such a thing was a very important part of being a successful runner.

So when, in the weeks after the Veteran's Memorial 5K, that seasonal depression reared its ugly head, my running severely slacked off. Pretty much to the point of nonexistence. It was September and I still had two 5Ks scheduled for the remainder of 2012—one in October and one in November—but between those races I wasn't doing much running. I'd lost my mojo and I was honestly starting to worry I'd never get it back. Even after those October and November races, I still had to contend with winter. If I couldn't even manage to get out and run when it was still relatively nice out, how on earth was I going to get through the cold, dark days of December and January?

What I needed was a big push, something to encourage me and keep me motivated enough to keep running. Something that would inspire me to keep going, to run towards a better version of myself.

Then, like fate arriving in the form of an email, I was notified that in 2013 the Rock 'N' Roll Marathon series was coming to the home of Rock 'N' Roll for an inaugural event.

Despite the name, the Rock 'N' Roll races cover the spectrum of distances, from 5K all the way up to the full marathon. The race offerings depend entirely on the city, with some offering the smaller races and others not. These destinations—or "Tour Stops" as they are known—cross international waters and runners who travel and participate in multiple races can earn extra medals beyond the usual finisher's bling.

Cleveland was getting a half marathon in the fall, which was basically the seasonal opposite of the officially named Cleveland Marathon held annually in May. While the Cleveland Marathon is local and more grassroots, the Rock 'N' Roll Marathon series scales the globe, bringing with it a name recognition that few other races can claim.

I sat at my desk, staring at the email, speechless. My mind started to move at warp speed as I considered the possibility.

Here I was, actually contemplating running a half marathon.

I'd only been running for about six months and 3.1 miles was the longest distance I had yet tackled. Could I really add on another *ten miles* and be successful? Never mind being successful, could I physically run 13.1 miles and live to tell the tale? Was my body even capable of that?

13.1 miles. I mean, that's a long way to travel by foot. I live about ten miles from my job and, *lemme tell ya*, Monday mornings when nobody wants to be headed into work and everyone is in need of extra coffee, that commute in my car seems to go on forever. So to run above and beyond that . . . I wasn't sure that was something I could really do.

Well, I mean, *obviously*, at the time I was considering registering, it *wasn't* something I could do. Hell, I don't think I could have *walked* thirteen miles, let alone run them. The only people I know who can wake up on a Saturday and decide to go run thirteen miles with very little training are ultra-marathoners. Those people who run fifty or hundred miles for a single race. To them, thirteen miles is like three to me.

Perspective, baby. It's all about that perspective.

Once that seed was planted, once the idea of running a half marathon entered my brain, I started to consider the possibility. There were just some logistical things that needed to be figured out first.

Mainly, it's important to note that half marathons are not cheap. Up until this point, the most I'd paid to register for a race was maybe $30 and even that probably included online processing fees, with the actual registration cost only being $25.

Now, though, I was looking at paying over $100. For me (and for most non-billionaires), that's not a small chunk of change. Also, the registration was both nontransferable and non-refundable. If something happened—I got injured, my training didn't go so well, family emergency, whatever—I'd be out a hundred bucks and not even have a fancy finisher's medal to show for it.

This was a big decision I was about to make. Both physically and financially. And there was no guarantee I'd be able to do it. Before registering for the my first 5K, I'd already run three miles, which meant that when I started to fill out the online registration form and input my information and credit card number, I was already confident in my abilities to complete the distance on race day.

But with this . . . running 13.1 miles before signing up, just to make sure this was a feasible endeavor, wasn't an option. This had to be done on blind faith.

I'm a fairly risk-adverse individual. I don't like failing—not that anyone does—but I make a point to not take chances unless I'm pretty confident in my abilities and the end result. On the flip side of that, when I am confident I'm tenacious as hell. When I know what I want—and I know I can get it—I'm not afraid to go after it and do whatever it takes.

That was the place I was in now, reading over the information about the Rock 'N' Roll Cleveland Half Marathon.

The risk-adverse gene in me was pointing out the financial and physical strain I'd be putting on my wallet and my body, with no way of knowing how I'd fare. It's not that I was concerned with my pace or place or any of that, but *could* I actually run 13.1 miles?

I know the saying goes "If I can do it, anybody can do it," but I don't know how much of that I believe. In real life, everybody is different and every *body* is different and maybe not every body is equipped to navigate the same endeavors, and that's okay.

Fear can be a paralyzer. Not so much fear itself, more the fear of the unknown. It's that whole risk-adverse personality. Without knowing if I'd be successful, if I'd cross that finish line in triumph, that fear started to creep in, leading to a sense of inertia.

Inertia, it turns out, is not that much different than ennui.

But that sense of dissatisfaction, of wanting and needing more and being unable to find it, is exactly why and how I ended up on the registration page for a half marathon. That ennui led me here—was I now going to stop short and not follow through merely because I didn't know what this would look like on the other side?

Once I registered, that was it. There was no turning back.

On the other side of the argument, though, is that if I planned on running this—if I followed through on registering, well over a year in advance of the actual race—I'd have that on the horizon. I couldn't just slack off my running and give into my fitness languor. I'd have to at least *try* and be consistent with my workouts.

Considering the planet Earth is four and a half billion years old, I recognize that twenty seconds doesn't seem like much in the grand scheme of things. After all, what all can a person really accomplish in such a brief amount of time? But like Chuck Palahniuk wrote in his novel *Rant,* "The future you have tomorrow won't be the same future you had yesterday."

As it turns out, with just a few keystrokes on the computer, twenty seconds is just long enough to entirely alter the course of your life.

In October, I ran the Nature's Bin 5K, a race that supported a local health food store. The race itself was in the nearby city of Lakewood with the start and finish line both at the beautiful Lakewood Park, overlooking Lake Erie and the city skyline off in the horizon.

The following month, I ran the Next Step Run for Shelter 5K at Edgewater Park. It was here that I won my very first medal. Granted, it was for fundraising, but that $1,065 I raised went towards helping homeless and underprivileged youth find a steady place of shelter. Not only was it the first medal I won—earned, not given—but it was my first medal ever. Considering my speed, it's unlikely I'll ever win any other kind of racing medal anytime soon, but that fundraising took a different kind of hard work.

It was now nearing the very end of 2012 and already my 2013 racing calendar was starting to take shape. But the Rock 'N' Roll Cleveland Half Marathon was still about a year away so I needed races to fill in the twelve months or so I had until race day.

Soon, my weekends were spent researching local races and I thought I had settled on a particular March race to be my first of the year, until my Uncle Don from Texas invited me down to run a race with him.

Now my uncle truly is a runner. The kind of runner who often wins awards in his age group. I'm fairly certain I'll never win an award in my age group unless I'm, like, eighty, and the only one that old still crazy enough to be running.

My Aunt Marianne had been in Cleveland over the summer and she first initiated the conversation about me coming down to Houston for a visit and to run with my uncle. She told him I thought that it sounded great and so he gathered a list of late winter and early spring races which he emailed to me with the instruction to pick one.

Living in Northeast Ohio, I'm accustomed to a racing schedule that follows the seasons. Ohio has all four seasons and that tends to determine the availability of races more than anything else. The calendar year is bookmarked by a small smattering of 5Ks and the rare 10K races in the very early and very late months of the year, with most races happening during spring, summer, and fall. Larger races in particular, the half, full, and ultra marathons, occur when the weather is on the warmer side.

Then there are cities like Houston. Cities that don't suffer from the inclement weather of the Midwest, but have a different weather problem.

To give some background, my mom grew up in the northern half of the United States and her parents relocated to Houston during the oil boom when my grandfather, an employee of Shell Oil, was transferred there. She was college-aged at the time and never really lived there except on breaks and so considers Ohio home, as does my dad.

When it came time to meet her parents, he traveled to Houston one summer. That was the first and the last time my dad went to Texas during that time of year because it was just too damn hot. The doors from the airport open and the humidity hits you like a wall.

Many Houston races are held in the winter. Or well, they hold races during that season of snow that the rest of us call winter and they call slightly less hot.

I looked through the list of races that my uncle had sent me. All of them were held in February or March and after doing a bit of preliminary research on each one (i.e. Googling their website), I decided on the ConocoPhillips Rodeo Run. I mean, if I'm going to travel all the way to *Texas* to run a race, I might as well make the most of it.

Go big or go home, *amirite?*

Now came the hard part.

The ConocoPhillips Rodeo Run offered two distances: a competitive 10K and a noncompetitive (also known as a fun run) 5K. I had started running back in February. It was now November, which means I'd been running less than a year at the time.

By now I had completed five 5Ks. I was comfortable with the distance, but I also knew I had to be careful to not get *too* comfortable with it. Like the Rock 'N' Roll Half Marathon, this might be an opportunity to challenge myself to bigger and better things.

I told my uncle we should do the 10K.

In the moment, I was totally confident with that decision. But soon after, facing the prospect of traveling just over six miles via my not-so-speedy feet, I was feeling very overwhelmed and *very* unprepared. I knew that before I did anything else, I needed to find an appropriate training plan.

All of my previous races up to this point had been 5Ks and none of them had been completed with any sort of formal training plan in place. Oh sure, I used the Couch to 5K program as a guide, but I didn't really set out with an end goal. My first 5K at the Cleveland Metroparks Zoo just sort of happened and after that it was more of a self-fulfilling prophecy sort of thing: I knew I'd be able to finish the second 5K because I'd already finished one. And after finishing two, I knew I'd be able to finish the third because I'd already done two. I was pretty much running on sheer faith in my previous abilities more than anything else. Maybe not the smartest way to go about it, but sometimes it's just a matter of what it takes to get across that finish line on race day.

With this, I knew I needed some guidance in place to steer me in the right direction. A 10K was double my longest racing distance thus far and while at first I may have thought that because I could run a 5K I could easily run a 10K, now that I had to, y'know, think about actually running said 10K my confidence was a little less secure. Now that my bravado had worn off and I was left not entirely convinced this was something I'd be able to do, I knew I definitely required a plan to get me to where I needed to go.

Not knowing where else to start, I began looking around online for a 10K training plan and was daunted by the sheer number available. More than that, each one was unique in its own way and full of a dictionary's worth of phrases that were so unfamiliar it was as if I was reading a foreign language: Fartlek. Tempo run. Hill repeats. Granted, the last one was easy enough to figure out on my own, but the rest I had absolutely no idea. Then there were the speed workouts that looked like a complicated math equation worthy of Mensa. Things like 12 to 16 x 400m with a 200m jog.

What did that even mean? Was it even English? Furthermore, what on earth had I gotten myself into? I mean, I just wanted to *run*.

After what felt like weeks of random web searches I stumbled across a six-week 10K Beginner Training Plan on the website of the Boston Athletic Association.

The B.A.A. has been around since the late nineteenth century and is in charge of the esteemed Boston Marathon, the world's oldest and most competitive annual marathon. When I say oldest, I emphasize the *old* part: the Boston Athletic Association itself has been around since 1887 and its pinnacle racing event premiered in 1897. The Boston Marathon is so well-regarded by those in the know, it doesn't even need the "marathon" in the title. If ever in a conversation with a fellow runner, just say *Boston* and they'll understand.

So, what I'm basically saying, is that Boston is like the Madonna of the racing world. Or the Cher. Or the Adele. Or, well, you get the idea.

If I was going to trust anyone to get me across the finish line of my very first 10K, this seemed like the racing organization to go with.

In preparing for all of my previous races, I'd usually just run a couple of times the week leading up to race day and then just show up to the starting line and run. Fitting runs in around my work schedule didn't pose much of a problem, but now I had to make sure I carved out time to run and stay on top of my training.

Like most beginner or novice training plans, the one offered by the Boston Athletic Association had one goal in mind: to get the runner across the finish line of their very first 10K in one piece. That might sound kind of silly and simplistic, but when conquering a new distance, the mere act of finishing is a worthy and lofty goal and should be treated with as much respect and reverence as the time goals more advanced runners set.

This particular plan—one of several beginner 10K plans available on the B.A.A. website—was time-based, not distance-based. So instead of being directed to run two or three miles, I was directed to run 15 to 25 minutes, with the duration of each run increasing week to week.

At a glance, this is a fantastic way to design a running program since it's focused on increasing a runner's endurance. By slowly and methodically increasing the length of time a runner is running, the plan is able to naturally build up running stamina. Being a long-distance runner is one of those situations where tenacity tends to win out over speed because at the end of the day, it doesn't really matter how fast a runner is if they don't have the strength to maintain that pace for a long period of time.

The problem, of course, is that these time-based training programs are designed with a certain type of runner in mind. For me, in 25 minutes I can *maybe* get two miles in if I'm having a good day. Like a really good day. Like the kind of good day that a pop singer can make millions off of thanks to that one catchy summer song that waxes poetic about said really good day.

The B.A.A. beginner training plan capped out with a 50- to 60-minute run. With my speed, that translated to roughly four miles.

So essentially, for me, the flaw with time-based training programs is that I have absolutely no idea how much I "should" be running in the weeks leading up to the race. With a distance-based plan I know that my long run this week is three miles and in a couple of weeks it will be five miles. As a slow runner, I just know that 60 minutes is not enough time to cover what feels like should be a significant amount of ground a week before race day.

6.2 miles didn't seem like a tremendously far distance until I had to run it.

It's funny, really, how running has altered my perception of certain distances. 6.2 miles in a car feels like nothing and the first time I had a commute that was roughly the same distance as a half marathon I was thrilled, because it was the shortest drive to work I'd had in years. On the flip side of that, though, there was a period in my life when my twenty-mile commute felt like it was the longest route ever and I couldn't imagine running that amount of terrain let alone tacking on an additional six-plus miles and running a full marathon.

With a training plan selected and in place, I now had to actually start training for my race. There was just one little, tiny detail I had sort of conveniently forgotten when I decided to run a 10K in February: training in the winter. In Cleveland.

<center>~~~</center>

When I first started running a year prior, I utilized the treadmill because I didn't really have any other options. But I was only running two or three times a week for a maximum of maybe thirty minutes at a time. Given the weather outside, this was really my only choice, although it wouldn't have been my first choice because the Treadmill is a loathsome creature.

Most people who hate the treadmill probably feel that way from some inherent, instinctual sense of self-preservation that tells them they should stay far, far away from that unnatural monster. I, however, come to my aversion the hard way. I have come face to face with the beast on the battlefield. I have stared down into its black belly and have seen its dark soul and have the scars to prove it.

Shortly after graduating college with my BFA in Creative Writing,

I moved back home (because, hi, I have a BFA in Creative Writing) and was once again living with my parents. I had a job. Well, I had two of them, which meant I was working six days a week. Evenings and weekends were my time to decompress and chill, which usually resulted in me binge-watching *Grey's Anatomy* and *Lost*. (Keep in mind, that this was before Netflix and to do said binge-watching, I had to get in my car and drive to the video store, and woe was me if someone else was binge-watching the same show and got to the video store for the next sequence of DVDs before I did.)

My mother, ever watchful, realized I was getting myself into a cycle where I would spend my days sitting in an office in front of a computer and then come home and spend my evenings sitting in my bedroom in front of a television screen. We had a gym down the street that my dad had been a member of for years, and my sister and I had occasionally gone there as children to swim laps in the pool or pretend we knew what we were doing with a racquetball.

Because they didn't want me to spend all of my free time draped across furniture in a nearly catatonic state, my mom encouraged me to get a membership to the very same gym and even sweetened the pot by offering to pay for it for me.

Well, hell. I mean, I didn't really have an excuse at this point to say no, now did I?

The gym was by far the nicest facility I'd ever seen, though I really only had my outdated college recreation center for comparison. There was a pool, racquetball courts, saunas, an indoor walking/running track, and fancy locker rooms. When I checked in they gave me a towel and it was just so damn *fancy*.

There were also machines. Lots of machines. On the far side of the building was the cardio equipment, which was comprised of various machines like ellipticals, stair climbers, and, yes, treadmills. Lots of treadmills. A whole long row of them in fact, right up against the half wall that divided the sunken equipment room from the indoor track. Being someone who enjoyed walking, that's what I would do on the treadmills. Sometimes I'd use the indoor track, but mostly I'd only hop on the treadmill since that's where the televisions were.

Being that this was a good almost fifteen years ago, I didn't have a fancy iPhone or iPod that held an entire lifetime of music (including, naturally, my beloved Barbra Streisand). No, I had a Discman, which allowed me to only listen to one CD at a time, meaning that I had to go to the gym prepared.

The thing about Discmans is that they are big and bulky. They are made to fit CDs, which, while not big and bulky per se, are obviously not as slim and sleek as a simple MP3 file. Well, okay, so CDs are slim but they are also wide and the Discman needed to be even wider. These days when I go running I can just pop my iPhone into my armband or tuck it into a pocket in my jacket or easily prop it on the elliptical dashboard.

Not so easy with the Discman, which I'd have to sort of awkwardly put into the cup holder on the treadmill and hope I didn't accidentally tug at it while fiddling around with my headphones and cause it to fall.

Which, of course, means that one day I was fiddling around with my headphones and pulled the Discman from the precarious safety of its cubby and it tumbled down onto the treadmill's moving belt.

Instinctively, I reached down to pick it up. Because that's what you do when a relatively expensive personal electronic goes falling towards the floor: you reach for it.

Most of the time, I advise people to trust their instincts. If your gut tells you to do something, you should probably do it. The asterisk to that advice is that if you are on a fully operational and currently running treadmill and your musical device falls, you should probably just let it fall. At the very most, you should turn the treadmill off before attempting to retrieve it. At the very least, move your feet to the stable sides of the belt while deciding your next course of action.

I did none of these things.

Nope, all I did was reach down for the Discman while still walking on the treadmill. This caused my balance to shift on the moving belt and while it wasn't moving very fast, it was still moving. In turn, I then lost *all* of my balance and slid down the length of the treadmill to the very end and onto the floor, the belt still moving.

At many other gyms, this would probably be nothing more than a silly little story where I stood up, shook myself off, laughed at my stupidity, and got back on.

If that were the case, though, I probably wouldn't be writing about it.

See, this row of treadmills was situated in front of a wall that divided the equipment from the indoor track. The gap between said treadmill and the wall was just wide enough for a person to walk up onto the treadmill. A gap that I was now stuck in between.

So there I was, pinned between the wall and the running treadmill, my arm up against the moving belt, which, again, wasn't moving very fast, but was *still moving* and now moving against the exposed flesh of my arm.

Three miles per hour when you're walking doesn't feel very fast. Three miles per hour on a treadmill, though, translated to a friction burn feels like Usain Bolt in the middle of a 100m sprint with my arm as the course.

Years ago, I read Stephen King's short story collection *Everything's Eventual*, which opens with the story "Autopsy Room Four." In it, the protagonist Howard wakes up from an unconscious state only to find himself on a table in the morgue. The doctors think he is dead and Howard, paralyzed but fully aware of what is happening, is struggling to communicate with them before they start the autopsy proceedings but is unable to get through.

As much as I utterly adore Stephen King's writing, there are few things worse in life than the terror of feeling like a character in one of his stories.

In the fetal position on the floor in the far back of the equipment area, tucked behind all of the machines, I was pretty much out of sight of everyone. But I could see them and my eyes followed them, willing one of them to look in my direction. Terrifying doesn't begin to describe it. I thought I called for help. I distinctly *remember* calling for help. But it may have all been in my head, like the internal screaming of a paralyzed patient living in the nightmares and dreamscapes of the master of horror, because when I was finally spotted and one of the employees came running over to rescue me, the first thing he asked was why I didn't yell for help.

Panic makes time crawl and it's entirely possible I was only there for a minute or two, and not the five or ten it felt like, but it was long enough for the treadmill belt to rub my arm raw. It was pink and red and throbbing for months, then orange and brown and scabbing for months.

I spent the entire summer in long sleeves.

Some people say they hate the treadmill because it's boring and the runners don't go anywhere and there's no change in scenery and they can't run as fast indoors as they can outdoors. Granted, I've said all those things, too, but my fierce loathing goes much deeper than that. Because when *I* say I hate the treadmill or when I say that I've had bad experiences with that particular exercise machine, that's the kind of evil shit I'm talking about.

Unfortunately it's also a necessary evil. Especially for runners living in a temperate climate like that of, say, Northeast Ohio. My training started in late January, with the ground outside my apartment covered in snow and ice. Running in snow is no joke and running on ice is even worse. It's not even just running: when I was in sixth grade I broke my left wrist after just walking on ice. (Okay, well, I wasn't walking so much as pretending to be an Olympic figure skater, only I wasn't wearing ice skates since I don't know how to skate. I was just wearing my boots on the frozen pond of one of those ritzy McMansions on the north side of town and I was twirling around and fell and slammed my wrist down on the ice and thus, a broken bone.)

But I might as well have been walking and if I managed to break a bone just doing that, there's no way I was going to risk another broken bone by trying to run on ice.

I had six weeks between now and my 10K. If I was going to train for this bad boy and train successfully, I was going to have to suck it up and meet my old foe yet again. With hard work, dedication, a training plan, and an arm sleeve for my fancy iPod, I was going to tackle this beast and I was going to win.

6

Everything's Bigger in Texas

Six weeks prior, I started following my first official training plan. There were early morning runs and late night workouts and sacrificed sleep. I had done my fair share of cross-training and strength training and, of course, running, all on that stupid, stupid dreadmill. Now, a month and a half later, I had finally arrived:

Race weekend.

The ConocoPhillips Rodeo Run 10K wasn't just going to be my very first 10K, this was also my first destination race. Which meant I had to travel to get to the race location. By airplane. Which meant packing. Which meant copious lists of what to take to make sure I had absolutely everything, and then packing and repacking multiple times just to make sure yet again that, no, I did not forget my shoes and, yes, they are packed in my carry-on because while I could handle my luggage being lost, I couldn't handle my shoes going missing into the airplane ether. So they were coming directly on board with me.

Amid all the packing I couldn't help but reflect on how far I'd come. Just one year ago I had been watching an episode of *The Biggest Loser,* overweight and out of shape. After witnessing the even more overweight and out-of-shape contestants run on the treadmill, I felt inspired enough to lace up a cheap, mostly new pair of running shoes that had been taking up space in my closet for years and hop on the treadmill myself.

Almost exactly 365 days later, I was about fifty pounds lighter and in the process of preparing to go run my first 10K race.

I had followed the Boston Athletic Association's novice 10K training plan as best I could. Physically, I felt completely prepared to tackle the distance ahead of me.

But mentally? Oof.

Mentally, I was seriously starting to question all of my life choices up until this very moment.

What really flummoxed me was that around the same time as when I had registered for this 10K, I had also signed up for a half marathon and I was weirdly feeling totally confident about those 13.1 miles.

But a 10K? Jesus, what the hell was I thinking getting myself into this?

So a 10K is double the distance of a 5K and a half marathon is basically double the distance of a 10K. Yet when I really tried to mentally see myself putting the work in and crossing those finish lines, all 13.1 miles of half marathon seemed far more of a realistic goal than a 10K and 6.2 miles.

Whiskey. Tango. Foxtrot.

I am a creature of habit. I have my routines, my levels of comfort. Stepping outside of those routines, coloring outside the proverbial lines, and challenging myself to be uncomfortable is, well, you know, *uncomfortable.* But it's a careful balancing act of reality and perception. For that reason alone, it would make more sense to believe that the challenge of running 13.1 miles would be far more daunting but because it was yet so out of reach, I had this somewhat romanticized view of what that would be like.

With a 10K, especially after nearly two months of training, it was a very, very real finish line I was closing in on and it left me terrified. I wasn't afraid of failing, because I knew I could do this. I was afraid of the very opposite: I was afraid of *succeeding*. Because once I set a new goal, once I raise the bar on my level of comfort, and then once I meet and *exceed* that bar, I can never go back. A new level of comfort will have been established.

Metaphor time: a caterpillar knows nothing else. He exists in his own little world, slowly inching and munching along leaves and branches, completely oblivious to anything outside his own realm of experience. There are probably other caterpillar friends and maybe even a family of caterpillars and they all are more than happy with the way things are in the gardens and trees where they live.

He's got a good life, that little caterpillar.

Then, one day, he wraps himself up into his tight little cocoon and a transformation begins to take shape. Things might be dark, maybe even a little scary, because the caterpillar's body is changing. He doesn't know what's happening, he's only sure that something deep inside him is working its way out. By the end of this transformation, he won't be the same little old caterpillar anymore.

Sure enough, one day, the cocoon breaks open and suddenly the caterpillar discovers he's *flying*. He doesn't have to crawl along the ground from tree to tree, he can float above the flowers of the field, his beautiful wings flapping in the wind. Who knew such extreme beauty had existed inside of him this whole time? And now, what *freedom* he had! After experiencing such liberation, he couldn't go back to his lowly life as a caterpillar again even if it was physically possible.

Which it isn't. Once that level of metamorphosis takes place, there's no way to return to the previous state, either mentally or emotionally.

In some ways, progressing through the hierarchy of race distances is kind of like life as the little caterpillar. Once the finish line of a new race is crossed and that distance has successfully been completed, a runner can't just go back to the start line and pretend it never happened. A runner can't un-run a race.

Not all runners want to increase their race distances. Some prefer the shorter 5K and have no desire to ever move up to a 10K or half, let alone a full marathon. But even then, once a runner tastes a certain speed, finishes within a certain time, achieves that PR, they can't take it back. That previous November, I had run the Next Step Run for

Shelter 5K, finishing in 41 minutes and 33 seconds with an average mile pace of 13:24. After finishing, I posted my time on social media and my cousin Matt, also a runner, commented that a 40-minute 5K would be next.

As I'm writing this, it's been almost five years and the Next Step Run for Shelter 5K is still my 5K Personal Record. I've run many, many 5Ks since, some with finish times that are close, others with times much slower. Even now, knowing a 13-minute mile, specifically three of them in a row, is unrealistic, I still show up at every 5K ready to chase that PR. Because when I ran that day, I literally felt like I was flying. Having felt that way once, I want to be able to feel it again. Once that PR has been set, all a runner can do is keep trying to beat it at every subsequent race.

So, in that way, that was what I found so terrifying about running the ConocoPhillips Rodeo Run 10K. It wasn't the distance itself, not really. I had trained, I had done my runs, and I knew that when I showed up at that start line, I'd be able to successfully cross that finish line at the end of the course.

It was what was on the other side of that finish line that scared me.

In the days leading up to the race I started to make a packing list, checking it twice. And three times. And four times. My shoes, as I said, were going in my carry-on because I had read horror stories about runners traveling for races who had packed their shoes in their luggage and gotten to their final destination only to discover that their suitcase did not. Everything that was packed in my suitcase, like my running clothes, could be easily and inexpensively replaced. But I was possessive about those running shoes, and the last thing I wanted to do was have to run my very first 10K in a new pair of shoes that hadn't yet been broken in. They were also bright pink, a shade of neon pink straight out of the 1980s, and the rest of my outfit was black which meant those pink shoes were gonna stand out for miles and there was no way I was gonna lose that photo op.

The race was Saturday morning but because of my work schedule, I didn't work Fridays, as well as the traditional weekend days. To take advantage of this and maximize my time with family, I was flying into Houston late Thursday night. My job itself was located close enough to the airport that I arranged my day to leave work a couple of hours early Thursday and drive straight to the airport.

Thanks to the time difference between Houston and Cleveland, I arrived in the early evening and was met at the airport by my Aunt Marianne and Uncle Don. They took me out to dinner at a local Italian restaurant in their neighborhood, then back to their house where I crawled, exhausted, into bed and fell asleep right away.

As I've said, most of my mom's family lives in Houston. At the time of the 2013 ConocoPhillips Rodeo Run 10K, this meant my Aunt Marianne, Uncle Don, Aunt Nancy, Uncle Steve, and my Grandma. Because of the 1,300-plus miles between Cleveland and Houston, I don't see them very often. I used to see them regularly when I was a kid, when my nuclear family would travel to Texas for Christmas— the end of December weather always being more preferable there than in Northeast Ohio—or when the Texas relatives would come to Ohio in the summer, mostly for the same seasonal reasons. But as my grandparents got older, travel for them became less convenient, and as my sister and I got older, our school and work schedules made it less convenient for us. So this particular late February weekend, along with the time for my first 10K, was also a bit of a family reunion.

Friday morning I woke up ready to run. The night before, over dinner, my Uncle Don suggested we go for a quick run in the morning. Just something short around their neighborhood. Partly to give our legs one final push before the race, but also to get me used to running in a much different climate.

Most of my training for this 10K had been indoors on the treadmill. Over the six weeks I had worked myself up to this distance, I wasn't given many opportunities to take my long runs outside so I was grateful for a chance to put my legs to work somewhere other than the treadmill. Houston in late February is like spring to me. Ohio in late February is like something out of *Dr. Zhivago*. Driving around the city, seeing the homes covered in snow with single-digit temperatures outside, it was impossible to not be reminded of that infamous ice palace scene. (February also usually meant that stupid groundhog out in Pennsylvania would predict another six more weeks of winter, not exactly helping matters.)

Running outdoors in Houston near the end of February is much different than running outdoors in Cleveland near the end of February. Back home, I had to contend with snow and ice and bitter winds in my face. In Houston, I was wearing a sleeveless shirt.

This was also an opportunity to get used to running with another person, side by side. Running is a solo sport for me. Everyone has his or her or zir preferences, of course, but I like the freedom that running alone gives me. I get to decide pace and the route.

Mostly, though, running by myself means I don't have to worry about my pace and its effect on another runner. Everyone has their own idea of what it means to be "slow," and more than once I've heard a slow runner quantify it by saying "I'm slow. Like, *really* slow." Hell, I've said that myself, and it almost always comes up with regards to running with another person, whether a race or just wanting to run in general.

That afternoon, after having lunch with my Grandma, my Uncle Don and I went to the local running store to pick up our packets.

This running store is located in a small shopping district surrounded by a bunch of other stores and earlier in the day my aunt had offered to take me shopping, just because. Well, really, it's because my aunt and uncle don't have kids, so my sister and I tend to benefit from this in unexpected ways.

I knew that when my Aunt Marianne made this offer she meant shopping for, say, a fun new dress to wear to dinner with the rest of my family the next night. But as we were walking around the store, I noticed a section off to the side that caught my interest.

I feel it necessary to update a previous statement I made earlier that the most important thing a runner can buy is a decent pair of shoes. While that's still true, there needs to be an amendment aimed at the women out there: *buy a good sports bra.*

It has already been established that math was not exactly the high point of my educational career and I frankly remember next to nothing from any of my classes. One thing I *do* remember is improper fractions. These are fractions where the top number is bigger than the bottom number. Something like 5/2 is an improper fraction, with 2½ being the proper form.

While learning about these fractions in fifth grade, the teacher told my class that another way to think about improper fractions is to call them Dolly Parton fractions because they are bigger on top.

Fifth grade. True story. Hard to forget improper fractions after that.

That being said, Dolly inspires another lesson here—who doesn't love Dolly, right? *Steel Magnolias, Nine to Five, Hannah Montana,* I mean the list goes on and on. My absolute favorite Dolly role ever is from the film *The Best Little Whorehouse in Texas,* a film I first saw when I was about fifteen or sixteen, which is really kind of awkward and borderline inappropriate, now that I think about it.

Anyway, there is a scene where Dolly's character Miss Mona is talking with Ed Earl (played by Burt Reynolds) about her former dream of being a ballerina dancer. Ed Earl, having a little bit of a crush on the madame of the Chicken Ranch, encourages Miss Mona to show off her dance moves. Miss Mona scoffs, saying, "Me jumpin' up and down? I'd black both my eyes!"

Running without a proper sports bra? Kind of like that.

Look, I don't want to get too graphic here but sometimes you just gotta strap that shit down, okay? I mean, unless you *want* to channel your inner lifeguard and look like someone who just stepped out of the opening credit sequence to *Baywatch*. In that case, be my guest. I'm not here to judge. You do you.

But for me, running around with boobs basically flying everywhere, unsupported, is uncomfortable as hell and it fucking *hurts* later, too. It's bad enough worrying about how my legs feel after a run, who the hell has time to worry about if my boobs are sore or not from all that excess and unnecessary bouncing? Boobs are not circus acts, people. They are not meant to fly through the air with the greatest of ease.

Strap. That. Shit. Down.

So there I am, standing in the middle of a running store with an aunt offering to buy me a fancy new frock just for fun and I'm eyeballing the very practical sports bra section of the store.

I had officially created a monster.

Glancing over at my aunt, I could tell this really wasn't at all what she had in mind so I allowed myself to be taken to Ann Taylor where I got a gorgeous dress that I looked absolutely divine in.

Sometimes you just have to pick your battles, *amirite?*

～～～

So here it was, the morning of my very first 10K; when they say everything is bigger in Texas, that includes races.

To be fair, I did pick a race centered on the annual rodeo and if you know anything about rodeos and/or the Lone Star State than you know that rodeos are a big fucking deal. So, naturally, the race associated with the 10K is an equally big fucking deal. Like, this was hard-core *legit*. On race day, 15,000 runners showed up to run either the 5K or the 10K. Those were the only distances being offered and 15,000 people showed up. That's like an entire small town. I've run in equally populous races, but not for distances short of a half marathon. For so many people to register for events of this distance speaks to the significance of this event.

That early in the morning there was a slight chill in the air, so I was glad I had brought along a fleece jacket that I wore while we stood around waiting. Downtown Houston was packed full of people, both with runners camped out near the start line, and with sidewalks jammed full of spectators ready to cheer us on. Somewhere in the mad mix was my Aunt Marianne.

Uncle Don and I made our way through the throng of people, attempting to find where all the runners were lined up. This race didn't have any official corrals for runners to utilize but they did have pacers standing among the other runners, signs with finish times and paces held high. We used those signs to figure out an appropriate place to stand and wait.

We lined up about 20 or so minutes before the start, but because there were so many people, there was a delay and it took us 10 minutes to get to the start line. By that time, the sun had come out and the Texas heat was starting to show. I knew there was no way I'd be able to run 6.2 miles wearing my fleece jacket.

Eventually it was our turn, as we finally made our way to the start line. As we crossed the blue mat that activated the blue chips on our shoes, I started my heart rate monitor. I wasn't wearing it to actively monitor my heart rate, but more so I'd have a general idea of our pace. I had a goal in mind and with the lag in clock and chip times, I couldn't use the clocks along the course to keep track but with the clock on the heart rate monitor I could.

Less than a quarter of a mile after we started, Uncle Don pointed out my Aunt Marianne standing on the sidelines. She was waving at us, clearly excited to spot us along the course. He and I quickly made our way to her spot on the sidewalk and passed off our jackets for safekeeping. We waved goodbye and carefully moved back into the flow of runners and set our sights on the finish line six miles away.

In our conversations leading up to race weekend, he and I discussed what our "running together" would look like. He's much faster than I am, but was willing to significantly slow down his pace at this race so as to match mine, which I greatly appreciated. But we also talked music and I said that while I usually always run listening to my iPod, I was okay with keeping the earphones and iPod tucked away.

And, at the start of the race, I totally was okay with that. He and I kept a pace that pushed us physically but still allowed for brief conversations. I was even okay with it through the first mile. After that, though, with that first mile marker crossed, I was becoming too *aware* of what I was doing.

Running is one of those things that actually sort of kind of sucks when you're in the middle of it. Not all the time: every once in a while I have a really great run, the kind where I'll run more than I planned or need to just because I don't want to stop. I always feel great after a run, but *during* . . . while running I am, more often than not, wondering why I took up running to begin with.

As long as I can get into that zone and close off the rest of the world and ignore what my body is doing, I'm capable of amazing feats. But if I'm too in the moment, too *aware* of what my body is doing, I tend to be well, too in the moment. Instead of focusing on the crowds and energy and other runners and internalizing all the awesome of race day, I instead focus on the negatives: Are my laces too tight? Too loose? My foot feels funny. Why does my foot feel funny? *WHY DOES MY FOOT FEEL FUNNY?*

Phantom pains. They are real. Especially on race day. Acknowledging and indulging them too much only seems to enable them to increase.

After only one mile, I could see my mind starting to work in that direction and with five miles still to go, I knew there was no way I could open up that part of my brain.

I turned to my uncle. "Would it be okay if I put my music on?"

He smiled and nodded, "Of course!"

I was so glad I had decided to bring my earphones and iPod, just in case. I pulled them out of my armband, popped the earbuds into my ears, and brought up my running play mix. I kept the music low enough that I could listen to the music, but still hear my uncle if he said something.

The race started downtown Houston, with the runners maneuvering around the large skyscrapers, and spectators cheering on the sidewalks. Around a mile and a half in, we passed a row of porta-potties set back off the road. My uncle said he was going to make a stop but that I should keep going and he'd meet up with him.

Temporarily alone, I plowed ahead and marveled at the city scape around me.

Because he's a fast runner, my uncle was able to quickly catch up with me again and we kept on running.

The course turned and veered onto the Allen Parkway, a highway that runs through downtown Houston. Like most highways, there is a median in the middle of the road. The course ran west along the Allen Parkway for a couple of miles before turning around and heading back towards downtown Houston.

As we ran along the Allen Parkway, my uncle caught my attention and gestured toward the other side of the median: there, running alone, was the eventual 10K winner, Sammy Kiplagat. He ran fierce and fast, his form flawless, and there was not a drop of body fat on his muscular frame.

Sammy is one of the "Kenyans," an elite group of professional runners that all come from the Republic of Kenya. Runners from Kenya are known throughout the sport as some of the best, especially in endurance races like half and full marathons. But, as evidenced by Sammy Kiplagat at the 2013 ConocoPhillips Rodeo Run 10K, they excel at shorter distances as well.

In the 30 minutes and 37 seconds it took Sammy to run those six miles, my uncle and I were just finishing up the first two. When it comes to out-and-back races—ones where the start and finish are generally in the same spot and the runners run for half the distance then turn around and head back towards the start area of the race— this is a familiar moment for me. I'll often see the elite and front of the pack already heading home only shortly after I start to gain some ground and get into my groove. But I don't run many races that attract runners of Sammy's caliber, so this was a first.

As we passed the Mile Two mark, I glanced down at my heart rate monitor to see how much time had passed. The heart rate monitor didn't give me a breakdown of my pace, but with some simple mental math gymnastics (even runners bad at math can do race splits in their head) I could figure out an average and ballpark how I was doing.

Noticing my movement, Uncle Don looked at me. "Is this pace okay?"

"Yup!" I said, grinning. "We're good!"

We had a plan going into this race. My uncle knew the Allen Parkway well enough to know that this was a very flat course. But there were some small dips along the way and my uncle suggested we walk the dips when they started to go back uphill. He also suggested we walk through the water stations. Considering my experience at the Running with a Mission 5K last summer and nearly choking on the water while trying to run and drink at the same time, I appreciated the suggestion.

I wasn't sure how I felt about walking during a road race, though. Walking almost felt like cheating in a way. Walking felt like it made me less of a runner.

But then I looked at my Uncle Don. This is a man who runs more frequently than I do and most decidedly runs faster than I do. He wasn't still trying to figure out what it means to be a runner, or find his identity within the world of racing. If he thought it was perfectly acceptable to walk during a race, then it was probably a good idea to listen to him and take him up on the idea. So, that's what we did: we ran, keeping a steady pace around a 14-minute mile, with brief walking breaks when we met a hill and also came to a water station. Which, y'know, is smart. Because the last thing I wanted was a repeat perfor- mance of my water drinking routine from my first 5K.

Physically, I felt strong and confident and I knew that my body would be able to keep up for the whole distance.

The mentally challenging part came around 3.2 miles. I was now in uncharted territory.

Miles are miles, sure. I certainly won't argue against that. But something about being in a race amplifies the importance of each mile marker you pass. Cleveland is a major metropolitan city, yes, but races tend to follow the same streets, streets that I live on and drive on, and, most importantly, run on.

I've gone running in a park or on a block that has been the location of a previous race and somehow the miles I ran in those races seemed to mean more than the miles I was running for fun. The commitment and level of dedication that comes with training for a race, eyes constantly kept on the prize, makes me feel the weight of those race miles, even if I've run that exact same route at a completely different time.

Mile 3.2 was now my longest racing distance yet, and I felt the importance of what it meant to run that distance and outstrip my previous comfort zone.

I was also halfway, which is always a bit of a double-edged sword. On the one hand you think *I'm already halfway.* On the other hand you often think, *Fuck, I'm only halfway.*

But even if I was in the latter frame of mind, what was I going to do? Quit? Leave my uncle to run the rest of the race by himself while I went and joined my aunt on the sidelines? Fuck no. So I fought through the mental block, telling myself I could do this. I will do this. I *am* doing this.

Then, there it was: the Mile Four mark. Oh, how I had been looking forward to seeing that sign.

Reaching the Mile Four mark meant that I had officially pushed myself out of my comfort zone into a new zone. There was no turning back now; I had crossed the threshold from someone who only ran 5Ks to someone who was about to rock her first 10K. From here, the only thing that stood between me and that finish line was two miles. Two measly, easy-peasy miles. (Okay, 2.2 miles, but for the sake of simplicity I'll round down.)

When running new and unfamiliar distances, it's sometimes mentally helpful to break that big distance into smaller chunks. Hell,

90

this is helpful even with old and familiar distances. Instead of focusing on the entirety of 3.1, or 6.2, or 13.1, or 26.2 or any and all distances above, below, and beyond, break it down into more manageable chunks. Even now I am sometimes overwhelmed by races distances, even ones I have completed multiple times, so I don't look ahead to the whole length of road standing between me and the finish line because it can be daunting.

At that first 10K, those 6.2 miles were overwhelming and daunting but instead of focusing on that, I set smaller goals. The first mini goal was getting to that initial 5K. That was a distance I was comfortable and familiar with. Then I pushed myself to get to Mile Four. After that, I just kept repeating to myself, *There's only two miles left. That's it, just two little old miles left.* I was like Dory over here: just keep running, just keep running. Two miles became one and a half, which became one, and before I knew it, that finish line was within sight.

Uncle Don and I stayed steady as we ran the last few yards of the Allen Parkway, wanting to finish strong. As soon as we crossed the finish line, we turned towards each other and embraced. My official time was 1:26, well within my 90-minute goal.

We exited the course and went to the small finisher's village that ran on a parallel road. Right at the exit of the race we were able to get some post-race nourishment, including bananas and chocolate milk. The rest of the road was full of tents represented by local organizations and some smaller national brands, handing out free swag and samples.

Soon, my Aunt Marianne found us and gave us both hugs and snapped a quick picture. She was still holding my black fleece jacket. As soon as I saw it I realized I was freezing—it's a natural reaction the body goes through after a hard workout, when the heart rates comes down. The finisher's village was under a long shade of trees, which only increased the cold sensations as my body started to recover from running over six miles. My aunt gave me back my jacket and I immediately put it on, wrapping myself tight in an effort to warm up.

As I put it on, I noticed the red pallor of my skin.

The day had started out chilly and overcast, but after an hour and a half of running outside in the mid-morning Texas heat, I was not only drenched in sweat but had developed quite a lovely sunburn as well. In all my packing and preparation, it had not occurred to me that sunblock might be a good idea. After all, it was February and I had come from Northeast Ohio. Needing sunblock this time of year was nowhere in my thought process.

Oops.

If nothing else, at least I wasn't all pasty winter white anymore.

After visiting all of the booths in the finisher's village, the three of us started the long walk back to the car. I hardly noticed the distance, too amped up from having just completed my first 10K. Not only finished it, but hit my time goal with room to spare!

I spent the rest of the day with this kind of haze around me. I wanted to tell everyone I met about what I had accomplished that morning. The sense of pride was fierce with this one, let me tell you.

In the weeks and months leading up to the Rodeo Run 10K, I found myself almost paralyzed with fear, wondering and worrying about what I would find on the other side of that finish line. Because once I crossed it, I'd have made that transition from just a 5K runner to a runner who ran 10Ks and would soon be training for a half marathon and all sorts of other races beyond. Really, it was that whole concept of the beyond that freaked me out the most because once I crossed that blue mat laid out in the middle of a road in Houston, anything was possible. Once I crossed that line, there was no going back.

As I crawled into the back of my aunt and uncle's SUV and buckled my seatbelt, my eyes rested on the bright blue plastic timing strip still looped around my bright pink shoes. The same pink shoes that had just carried me across that finish line—both the actual finish line and the one in my head. Looking at that blue strip and knowing what it represented, I couldn't help but smile.

Turns out, I wouldn't have wanted to go back even if I could.

7
Eat, Sleep, Run, Repeat

The ConocoPhillips Rodeo Run 10K hadn't just been my first 10K; it had also been my first race of 2013. A few weeks later, in mid-March, I followed it up with the St. Malachi 5-Mile Run.

A Cleveland racing tradition as old as I am, St. Malachi itself is a well-regarded Catholic church with a long history within the community. So well known, in fact, that it used to appear on the labels of Great Lakes Brewing Company's Conway's Irish Ale, a seasonal beer that comes out in early spring. The race held in the church's honor is always held right around St. Patrick's Day, with a sea of green runners arriving to race the streets of Cleveland.

March weather in Northeast Ohio is incredibly unpredictable. Spring in general can be unpredictable, but March is a month of split personalities. With February, it's pretty much a given that there will be snow and most likely lots of it. Even when that groundhog over in our neighbor Pennsylvania predicts an early spring, there's still at least one more snowfall to deal with before that happens. By the time April rolls around, Clevelanders may still require a light jacket when they leave the house but there are still moments where things like flip-flops and Capri pants are reasonable without being underdressed.

For the 2013 St. Malachi race, the weather was far more akin to February than it was April. Snow, sleet, slush . . . if it was a cold and nasty form of precipitation that starts with the letter "s" that race had it. By the time I hit the water table at the halfway point, the water had been sitting in frigid temps for so long, the little waxy paper cups had ice crystals all around them.

Surprisingly, despite the weather, I ran slightly faster than I did at the ConocoPhillips Rodeo Run 10K. It's like my body knew the sooner I got to the finish line, the sooner I could get into a hot shower.

Two months later, I ran my second 10K, at home in Cleveland as part of the city's marathon weekend.

It was July by then, and with the change of seasons came a change in my running strategy. After spending the past six months running almost nearly one race a month, I was now cutting back on the number of races I ran. I had a much bigger finish line to chase.

It's 4:45 a.m. and there is a very loud, very annoying sound coming from the general direction of my nightstand. If I were a cartoon character, this is the part of the story where I would draw a huge hammer from beneath the covers and smash that alarm clock into a million thousand little pieces. There'd be springs and coils everywhere, the second hand making sad little half-tick attempts to continue its solitary job of marking time before it finally dies down, drooping over the broken face like a leftover from a botched Dali painting.

But I'm not a cartoon. I'm a runner and that shrill noise is my alarm clock. Keeping my eyes closed, I reach my hand out from under the warm space of my bed and into the cold space of my bedroom, groping across my nightstand in an attempt to find my alarm clock so I can shut the damn thing off.

Throwing the covers off, I will myself to sit up, eyes blurry, mind groggy. I stumble out of bed and start rooting around in the dark for my shoes, refusing to turn on the lights because my vision still needs to adjust and it's way too fucking early in the morning to try and shake myself awake. Dressing properly is already taken care of because I went to bed in my workout clothes. When it's this early and the gym is in my future, it's important to set myself up for success for actually getting to said gym and sometimes that means going to bed wearing a tech shirt.

Usually I am rather proud of the impressive rack I have been blessed with, but before coffee, often the logistics required to put on a sports bra capable of supporting it is a mental and physical challenge on par with a Mensa exam.

This is the fifth morning in as many days that I have woken up ridiculously early to workout before work. I wake up ridiculously early, then go work a long day, then come home and go to bed ridiculously early because—yay—tomorrow I get to yet again wake up ridiculously early and do it all over again.

It wasn't like this was my first go-around with early mornings and long days. Back in high school, my marching band had an opportunity to appear on live television as part of the Friday morning show for a local network. This meant being in place outside the studio by 5:30 a.m. For that to happen we had to leave our school by 4:30 a.m. and because we had a couple hundred people to organize onto buses, we were told to be at the school by 4 a.m. Our band director joked that the only four o'clock he thought existed was the one in the afternoon.

Oh, he was so clever that one.

After putting on a good show for the Northeast Ohio viewing area, we piled back onto our buses and went back to school, making it just in time for second period. Because, you know, we were students after all and our education was the priority. Then, because this was a Friday, we still had a football game to look forward to that night after school.

It kind of feels like that, only instead of it just being a one-time special event situation, it happens every day for several weeks or months in a row. Morning after morning, day after day, week after week. Worse, while we were told we had to attend the morning show, this exercise/torture routine that I had going was completely voluntarily.

Mondays: running. Tuesdays: spinning. Wednesdays: running. Thursdays: yoga. Fridays: running. Saturdays: running. Sundays: rest.

Welcome to training mode.

~~~

Ten months earlier I did something so out of character I still hadn't quite wrapped my head around it: *I had registered for a half marathon.* A half marathon that was now a mere two and a half months away. That's it, that's all that stood between me and 13.1 miles.

As a librarian by trade, I have a master's degree in Library and Information Science. I took multiple classes towards earning this degree that were spent focusing on the organization of information. Organization is my jam, man. This meant that when it came to selecting a training plan, I wasn't just going to follow that training plan. I was going to follow that training plan like nobody had ever followed a training plan ever before.

If I had learned anything from my training experience for the ConocoPhillips Rodeo Run 10K, it's that I like having a plan. I like to have structure, a guide to follow to constantly challenge myself. I like knowing that Mondays are for runs and Tuesdays are for spinning. Each day has a job, a mental focus. Something to concentrate my energy on, something to look forward to.

When it comes to plans, my brain works better if I can see the big plan. The long game. I printed out calendars for the next few months with each day's activity written in. These calendars got hung in my apartment in a spot that I would see every single day.

I loved being able to walk over and see what was on the agenda for the next day or the upcoming week. I loved being able to watch the progression of the long runs, slowly increasing with each new week.

But I especially loved being able to cross a day off after that particular activity had been completed. There was nothing more satisfying than taking a pen and drawing a diagonal line across the designated square on my calendar.

I had selected a well-rounded training program that included four days of running, two cross-training days, and a rest day.

Rest days are incredibly important to any training program as it gives the body an opportunity to rest (duh) and recover from all the hard work. But, as I quickly found out and as other runners can attest to, rest days are, oddly, one of the hardest days to get through.

Every morning, I was waking up early to lace up my shoes and run, or hop onto a stationary bike and spin, or contort my body into one of a dozen yoga poses. After all of that, instead of feeling restful on rest days I felt almost restless. I felt twitchy and fidgety, which surprised me tremendously. Normally I am a person who loves being lazy. Give me a comfy couch and a Netflix subscription and I'm good. After a morning run I fully indulged in lazy afternoons, but just resting for the sake of resting pushed me out of what was apparently my new comfort zone.

My body had gotten used to working out on an almost daily basis. More than that, it apparently *liked* working out that frequently, so when a rest day rolled around, it *wanted* to run more or spin more or find an even more difficult yoga pose. Having to chill and not exercise was challenging, even when I knew it was what my body needed.

My training runs were going well enough, although I was falling into the same trap I did last year: freaking out because the heat was slowing me down. When I had 6-, 7-, 8-mile runs on the agenda, I had to plan my days very carefully.

The previous summer, my runs had never gone beyond three miles, so I only had to find a sliver of time in my schedule (usually before work) to run. Now, though, because of the distance, I needed to carve out a substantial amount of time. Not only that, but with the heat I didn't have much flexibility with regards to *when* I started running.

When you live in a major city, it can take a lot of creativity to find places safe enough to run long distances and won't require stopping at an intersection every fifty feet.

This is where the Cleveland Metroparks once again comes into my story with its hundreds of miles of paved trails. As my training mileage increased, I decided to take advantage of all the local parks by trying out different ones when my Friday long run rolled around.

I'm already a naturally early riser but since adopting cats am even more so. While I am more than happy to sleep in until 9 or 10 a.m. every once in a while, my cats Chloe and Linus will not tolerate waiting that long for breakfast. (Well, Linus will, but once Chloe starts bugging me to wake up, he joins in. Because he apparently wants to be all cool like his big sister.)

So while Friday was a day off for me from work, I was usually up soon after sunrise, giving me plenty of time to run. Bonus: waking up early and knocking out my run first thing meant I still had the weekend ahead of me without having to worry about where to fit a run in.

But every once in a while, I do like to sleep in, so I'd forgo the early, early morning run for an extra hour or two of sleep. This was great and all until it is 10 a.m. and I'm only two miles into an 8-mile run and it's going to take me about another hour and a half to finish which means it's going to be closer to lunchtime by the time I'm done and it's already, like, a zillion degrees and OMG JUST KILL ME NOW.

Long stretches of the Cleveland Metroparks are shaded, but just as many are out in the open. Because people like sunshine or something. Which, sure, if it's a nice day in the summer and you're going for a walk I guess I can sort of appreciate being out and exposed like that. But when you're running for miles on end in the middle of summer, sunshine soon becomes The Enemy.

The weeks and months quickly passed and soon enough, the high heat of summer was passing and there was a slight chill in the air. With the drop in temperature, days were getting shorter: I no longer had as much daylight in the wee hours before work and the sun was beginning to set earlier each evening. When the thermometers start to dip, the mind naturally turns towards the months ahead: the red, orange, and gold leaves that would burst forth like flames of fire, gently abandoning their branches and falling to the ground. Soon there would be cool evenings full of warm apple cider and the basic girl heaven that is pumpkin spice everything and, eventually, snow finding the green grass and settling in among the blades, microscopic fields of crystals.

But I was getting ahead of myself. Before I could indulge in my most favorite season of all, I had to first finish my inaugural half marathon.

But before I could even do that, I had to finish my training plan.

When I first selected my training plan and mapped out all of the workouts and runs on my calendar, there was one particular run I was most anxious about, even way back in July.

As I learned in my research, many, if not most, training plans don't actually have a runner run the final, full distance until race day. The idea is that if a runner followed the training plan and kept up with the long runs then they should be well prepared for that full distance, even if they have never run it before. This isn't always true entirely across the board: some training plans do have runners not only run the race distance, some even go over on mileage, running fourteen or fifteen miles for a half marathon. Training plans like that, meeting the final distance before race day, are more often than not aimed at those runners chasing a time goal. I just wanted to finish no matter how long it took me.

I was following one of the training plans that did not go all the way up to 13.1 until the morning of my race. The term "long run" is a bit of a . . . well, not a misnomer exactly, but it is very dependent on perspective. All it really means is that it's the longest run in a week of training. For a 5K, long runs can be two or two and a half miles. For a 10K, four or five miles can suffice. For my half marathon training, my longest long run was ten miles.

Ten. Miles.

Toto, I don't think we're in the single digits anymore.

From the beginning of this whole running "experiment" (an experiment that was clearly by now less of an exception and more the rule), I was constantly finding myself lacking in confidence when it came to new distances. Running that first 5K, running that first 10K . . . each new race brought a new set of challenges. Challenges that I continued to meet and overcome.

Three miles? Easy. Six miles? Whatever. Nine miles? Eh, no problem.

But *ten* miles?

Whoa. Hold up here now and wait just a minute. What's this whole nonsense about running ten miles? What kind of people run ten miles? Don't they realize that's double digits category? I'll tell you what kind of people run ten miles—the kind of people who clearly don't have anything better to do on an otherwise gorgeous Friday morning in autumn.

People like me, apparently.

It was the middle of September, a time of year that is cool enough to require a light jacket. Especially first thing in the morning, which is my favorite time to run. It's my favorite time to run just as a general rule, but especially with a long run on the agenda. Because of my speed, I require more time to complete what others may consider quick runs. In this case, I was looking at close to three hours so the earlier I got out, the earlier I'd be finished, and the more time I'd have to relax and rest.

After waking up fairly early, I made a quick breakfast, knowing this distance was far too long to tackle on an empty stomach. I changed into my running clothes, put my shoes on, and added my hot pink running jacket, made of a lightweight stretchy material not unlike the tech shirts I sometimes get at races. Along with having a million pockets, inside and out, because it's so light, I don't worry about overheating when I start running. This is always an issue when I prepare to run in the cold and start to layer up—there will often come a point when I find I have clearly put on far too many layers but I'm pretty much stuck with whatever I'm wearing and have to suck it up until I'm done.

In recent weeks, I had started taking advantage of the over 20,000 acres that make up the Cleveland Metroparks, visiting various reservations and nature preserves around the area for a change of scenery. In fact, every Friday I'd look at the Cleveland Metroparks website and pick a new park or "reservation" to explore. This time, however, I wanted to keep things close to home so opted to return to nearby Edgewater Park.

The sky was overcast and grey, with large puffs of clouds blocking what little sun was available. Strong winds danced across the dark waters of Lake Erie, which had enough lift to cause waves. Brave surfers, unafraid of the biting temperatures, met the rising water with glee.

Edgewater is a multilevel park with a one-mile loop on the lower park and a roughly half-mile loop on the upper park. A somewhat steep incline that measures about a quarter of a mile connects the two loops. This meant that a full lap, upper and lower plus the hill, was less than two miles all around.

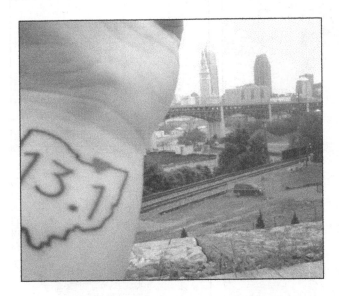

My half marathon tattoo against the Cleveland skyline.

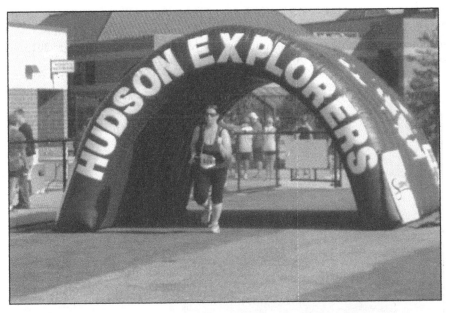

Veteran's Memorial Stadium. The girl who walked the mile in high school is running on the track as an adult! August 2012.

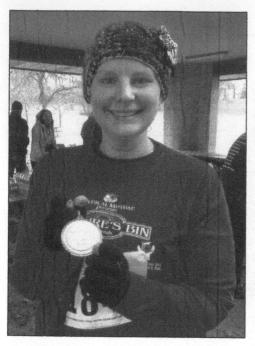

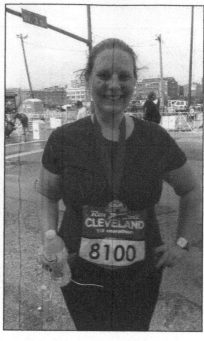

Next Step Run for Shelter 5K. I won the "Extra Mile Award" for raising the most money at the race. My 41:33 finish time is still my 5K PR. November 2012.

Rock 'N' Roll Cleveland Half Marathon. I am now a HALF-MARATHONER! October 2013.

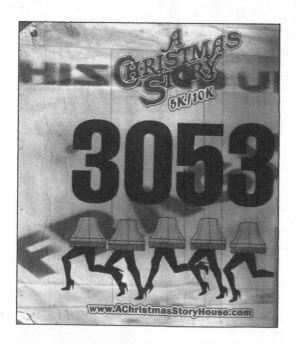

A Christmas Story 10K. Check out those running leg lamps on the race bib. December 2013.

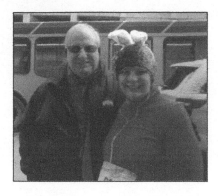

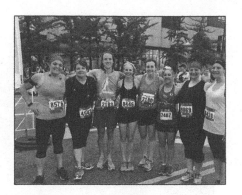

A Christmas Story 10K. My dad and I after I finished A Christmas Story 10K. Look at me dressed as the Pink Nightmare with the bunny ears! December 2013.

Rite Aid Cleveland Half Marathon. The Cleveland Marathon Ambassadors doing a pre-race photo op. May 2015.

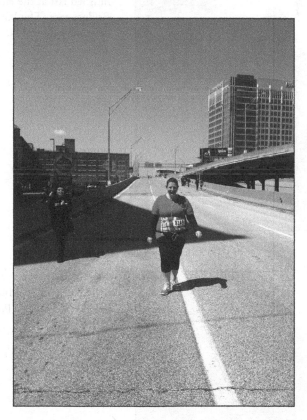

Rite Aid Cleveland Half Marathon. Walking down the Cleveland Shoreway ramp thanks to hurting my ankle at Mile Nine. May 2014.

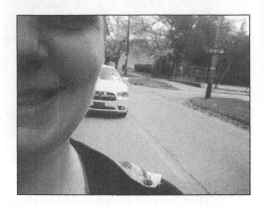

Running the Bridges. It's not last place—it's running with a police escort. November 2014.

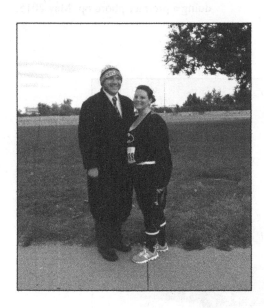

Running the Bridges. My boyfriend Ben and I after I finished last at the Running the Bridges race. The Batman costume held up! November 2014.

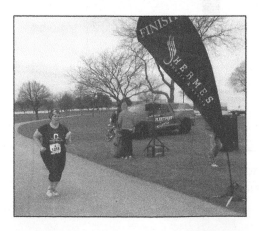

Cleveland 10 Miler. Finishing the Cleveland 10 Miler at my beloved Edgewater Park. April 2015.

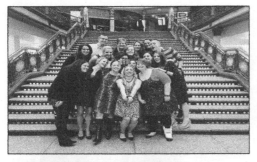

Rite Aid Cleveland Marathon weekend. The Cleveland Marathon Ambassadors at the VIP Reception. Look carefully and you can spot my air cast for my injured ankle. May 2016.

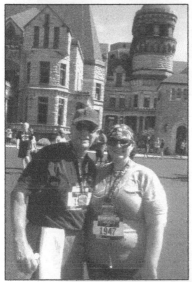

Shawshank Hustle. My dad and I in front of the old Ohio State Reformatory, filming location for *The Shawshank Redemption*. July 2015.

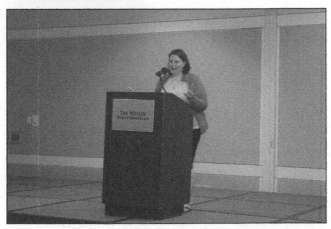

FitBloggin 2015. Presenting my Ignite! Fitness presentation at the FitBloggin 2015 conference in Denver, Colorado. July 2015. Photo Credit: Carrie D. Photography.

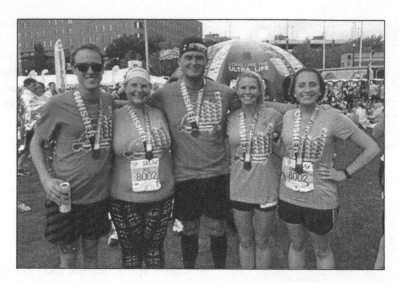

Akron Marathon Relay. The Tortoise and the Hares: Andrew, Me, Dan, Stephanie, and Melissa. September 2015. Photo Credit: Melissa Koski.

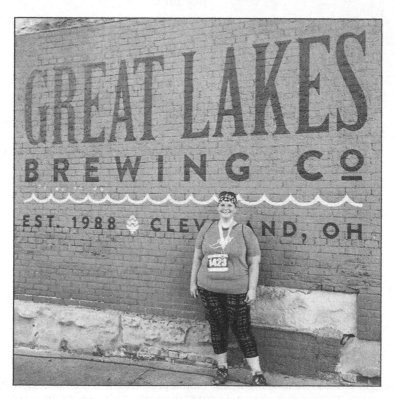

The Great Beer Chase 5K. After finishing the Great Beer Chase 5K, I *had* to pose in front of the Great Lakes Brewing Company wall. October 2015.

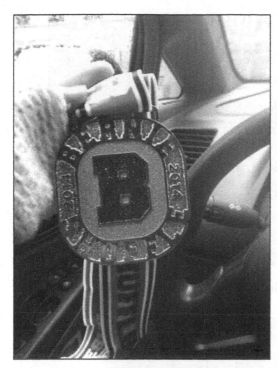

The Bernie Shuffle. Will Run for Bling. November 2014.

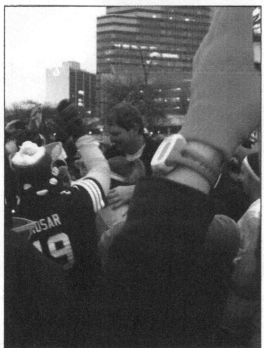

The Bernie Shuffle. Bernie Kosar and his fans at the start of the race. November 2014.

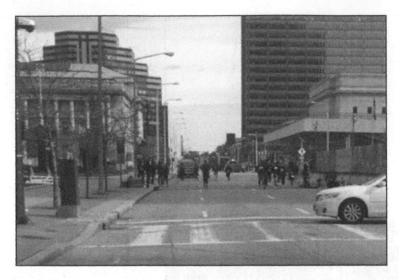

Cleveland Turkey Trot. Lackluster finish line at the Turkey Trot in November 2015.

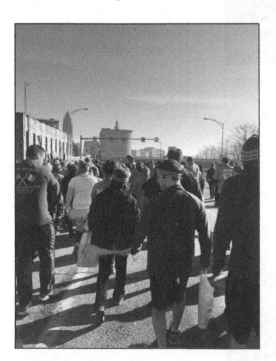

St. Malachi 2-Miler. A sea of green crossing the Detroit-Superior Bridge. March 2016.

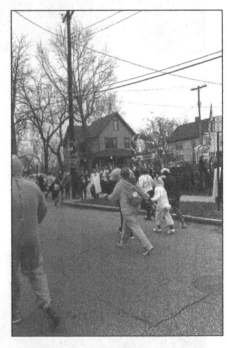

A Christmas Story 10K. Christmas Story House in the Tremont neighborhood, all decorated for the race. Lots of pink bunnies on the course. December 2015.

Running the lower lap is nice and easy, for no other reason than the fact that it measures almost exactly one mile all the way around. I was without a GPS watch and had to rely on my phone, a device that should have been upgraded years ago, so being able to accurately track my mileage was important.

That said, the thought of running ten laps around the lower loop bored me to tears just thinking about it.

Knowing myself well, if I got into a position where I was even the slightest bit bored while running I'd quit early, so I decided to set myself up for success by taking advantage of the park's topographical features and utilizing both the top and bottom loops. I decided to alternate: I'd run two loops on the bottom loop, then run up the hill and run a lap on the top loop. Then back down the hill only to do it over again.

Not only would I get some change in scenery and not have to view the same course for ten miles, I'd also get some hill work in as well. Because apparently along with running my longest distance to date, I hate myself enough to throw in some hills.

Runners really are masochists at heart.

I parked my car in the lot, then stepped out onto the lower level path and started running.

The air had that cold autumn bite to it and the wind coming off the lake was fierce and forceful. My decision to wear a jacket was clearly the right choice.

That particular Friday morning in September, Mother Nature was unable to make up her mind. Some moments I would see pockets of bright blue sky high up above, only to then lose the sun behind the clouds as the sky turned grey and overcast.

Several miles in, I started to feel small cold drops of water: it was sprinkling. *Please don't start to rain, please don't start to rain*, I repeated over and over again in my head. I don't mind running in rain and will do it if necessary. I mean, compared to the winter weather back in March that was the St. Malachi race, a little bit of rain is nothing.

But given the choice of running in rain or not running in rain, I will always pick not running in rain. Obviously.

It continued to sprinkle, but the impending storm held off long enough for me to finish my run. It took 2 hours, 43 minutes and at the end of it I was tired, cold, and drenched from a combination of sweat, rain, and Lake Erie spray.

But none of that mattered.

Because I had done it. I had done what was, without a doubt, the most badass thing I had ever done in my entire life: I had just run ten whole miles.

No, it wasn't a fast ten miles. Those ten miles took me almost three hours to complete. My average pace was over 16-minute miles. Other runners, faster runners, might boggle at being out there that long for "only" ten miles but for me, I felt like a running rock star.

Ten miles is ten miles, no matter how fast or slow it takes.

When I started training back in the summer, I spent all those weeks feeling anxious and apprehensive about this particular run. Physically and mentally I knew it would push me far beyond my comfort zone and challenge me in ways I couldn't even comprehend.

But I also knew that those ten miles would get me ten milers closer to achieving my goal of finishing a half marathon.

That was my last long run of my training plan. The Rock 'N' Roll Cleveland Half Marathon was still a few weeks away. From here I entered the tapering phase: tapering is the final part of a runner's training plan. During the last couple of weeks, a runner's training should focus less on running and more on resting, saving as much energy as possible for race day, while still staying loose and limber.

For many runners, myself included, tapering is the hardest part of the training plan. Harder than early morning runs, or long runs, or speed work, or all of the above. After weeks and months of working out on a near daily basis, suddenly runners are forced to, well, not workout and not run. At least not as often or as hard as they had been. The body is an incredible machine and it adapts quickly to a new schedule, a new lifestyle, and it starts to crave that new routine.

Tapering makes me twitchy. Like, there's really no other word for it. I have all this pent up energy that is just BURSTING to come out. Normally I can exercise as a means of alleviating some of it but not during tapering.

Really, it's like the meanest trick ever to play on a runner: oh here's a training plan. Go follow it, including all the early morning cross-training and the weekend long runs and training runs and this run and that run and just run, run, run and then BOOM. STOP. And not only do you have to stop, you have to stop right before the race. So now, my body, which is CRAVING the desire to run, is now feeling all twitchy and anxious because I have to cut back; and then I'm also feeling all twitchy and anxious because OH HELLO I HAVE THIS BIG UPCOMING RACE and, so, yeah. I don't like tapering.

The other thing tapering does is make you hungry as hell.

Getting "rungry" (see what I did there? Run + hungry) is a legit problem. It happens after normal training runs, too, which is why it's super dangerous to go grocery shopping after one. Oh, sure, you think you're fine. You get done with your run, it's still early enough on your day off, you decide to go pick up some groceries. You even managed to remember to bring your grocery list!

For the first half of the trip you're fine, you're picking up your produce and your fruit and vegetables. But then, suddenly, you find yourself in the cookie aisle. You don't even know how you got there, it's like your cart wandered over all by its little lonesome self. Just like those cookies managed to just jump off the shelf into the cart all on their own.

Same thing happens in the ice cream aisle. I don't know how that food does it.

When you're training, you can kinda sorta justify it by all that running you're doing (although, really, ice cream doesn't make the best pre- or post-race fuel) but then during tapering all of a sudden it's just FOOD FOOD FOOD. Like Cookie Monster, shoving those cookies in his mouth.

Ugh. It's the worst.

But at least I have those thirteen miles ahead that will maybe burn some of these calories off.

8

Lucky Number Thirteen (point one)

I imagine people of normal, healthy weights and body mass indexes watching those weight loss reality shows and wondering how people manage to get themselves up to weighing over 300, 400, or even 500 pounds. Maybe it doesn't even take a stranger on your television. Maybe it's the stranger you see standing in line at the grocery store, awkwardly having to step out into the main aisle to unload their groceries because the space between the conveyer belt and the snack shelf isn't wide enough for both them and the cart. Maybe you even peek into their cart and silently judge their food choices. Maybe it's the person you quickly jog pass as you hurry up the stairs while they huff and puff behind you, each step feeling insurmountable, a single staircase as challenging as climbing Mount Everest.

Speaking as someone who once weighed 311 pounds, I can tell you that it's really not that difficult. I ate a lot of food that's not good for me and is devoid of all nutritional value, and sat on my ass all day, watching other people lose weight on television. That's pretty easy.

As previously mentioned, my foray into running started back in late 2011 when my younger sister, Amy, sent me an email. In that email she expressed concern over my weight and health, concerned that she would lose her big sister to an early death.

I'd been dealing with similar comments from family for years but something about it coming from my little sister had the necessary impact and soon after I signed up for Weight Watchers Online. Doing it online meant I weighed in at home every week.

As it turns out, home bathroom scales only go up to a certain weight and I was too heavy for mine. I stepped on that old analog scale and watched the dial move around and around the numbers, unable to register my weight.

I couldn't remember the last time I weighed myself on that scale, but it had apparently been long enough to gain so much weight that it was no longer of use to me. I had to go out and buy a brand new digital scale that would be able to handle my weight.

If not for my sister and her email, I don't know if I would have had the courage to step on that scale to begin with and start the journey to lose weight.

I couldn't help but think about that email as I stood in my corral in front of the Rock & Roll Hall of Fame and Museum. Being that it was October, all of us runners were lining up when it was still dark out and as the sun started to rise, the rays bounced off the panes of the glass pyramid that anchors the museum.

I couldn't help thinking about it because in just a couple of hours I was going to be crossing the finish line of my very first half marathon. In that corral, surrounded by all the other runners, bouncing in place to try and keep warm in the early morning autumn morning I realized that 13.1—the amount of miles I was about to run—is the same inverted numbers as 311: my starting high weight.

If that isn't poetic, I don't know what is.

~~~

When I first registered for the race over a year ago, I had put down an estimated finish time of 3 hours. As I worked through my training plan it became clear that I wouldn't be able to keep up my normal pace over such a long distance and that my finish time was going to be closer to 3:30 so that's what I was aiming for when the gun went off and we started running.

The Rock 'N' Roll Marathon series is unique in that it sets up bands along the course who play live music, which was a nice motivator along the way. They were mostly local bands, set up close to every mile marker.

After the start at the Rock & Roll Hall of Fame and Museum, the course went slightly east for a few blocks before turning a corner and heading back west across the Cuyahoga River. Around the Mile Three mark, the course ran past my apartment building, which also brought along the first of two hills.

For once I was actually prepared—a few days before, when I ventured to the Cleveland Convention Center for the Expo—there was a video that took runners right along the course from the point of view of a dash cam. So I not only knew there would be hills, I knew exactly where they would be.

The Rock 'N' Roll series was prepared too, planting inspiration signs along the hills as well. My favorite said *Sweat like a pig, look like a fox.*

Wise words indeed.

Coming up the hill, the course turned onto Detroit, one of the major roads which runs through Cleveland's West Side. After running forty city blocks, the course turned down Franklin and headed back towards the city.

After passing the course marker for Mile Seven, I took a quick second to look down at my heart rate monitor. 10:20 a.m. When I realized that the race would take me right down the street where many of my friends live, I did some calculations and predicted I'd be coming their way between 10:15 and 10:45, depending on (a) what time I got out of my corral and started running, and (b) my pace.

I was right on schedule.

As I turned the corner from Abbey onto West 14th Street, my eyes were looking up and over, towards Missy's balcony. Many, if not most, of the single family homes in Tremont have been turned into apartment buildings and my friends had all found apartments in the same single block.

I was hot, I was tired, and I was only halfway through my first half marathon. If there was a moment when I needed some positive reinforcement to keep going, this was it.

From her balcony on the second floor of a barn red home, Missy waved and called my name. A homemade poster was attached to the railing. As I passed in front of her house I happened to glance down and saw a series of messages written in chalk on the street, my favorite being *Jilly-Bean! You Go Girl!*

My friend Lauren, having to work the day of the race, had gone out the night before and written the encouraging words of support for this very moment.

Now grinning and with a renewed sense of energy, I waved goodbye to Missy and kept chugging along through the next several miles.

I had done well for the past eleven miles of the race but here I was, with two miles or so to go, and I was starting to lose a little steam. Running was become less and less easy, not helped at all by the blisters I was starting to develop, and by the time the course reached the Lorain-Carnegie Bridge and was headed back towards downtown, I was walking more than running.

I was about halfway across the bridge when the racing van pulled up beside me and the driver asked if I was okay.

It's an interesting question to ask a runner right near the end of a long-distance race, *Are you okay?* I'm a fair-skinned natural blonde who had spent the better part of her morning exposed to sun, making my face pretty much match the fake red hair I've been sporting for over a decade. I also am one of those women blessed (or cursed) with overactive sweat glands. Some women claim to "glow" when they work out. I make no euphemisms. I sweat. Hard. Join me in spinning, or yoga, or Zumba, and by the end of class I will look like I have just taken a shower, with my hair soaked all the way through.

So I'm sweaty and beet red and I certainly don't look like a woman who should, traditionally speaking, even be running a half marathon at all. I was also walking slowly and perhaps a little funny thanks to the blisters.

When that driver asked me if I was okay, I knew that he wasn't just checking up on me—he was offering his services. The services that would entail me putting my tired tail between my legs, climbing into his van, and allowing myself to be driven the two more miles it would take to get to the finish line.

When he asked me if I was okay, I'd already been out there for close to three and a half hours. The majority of runners had finished hours ago and at this point in the day were probably having a big brunch and on their second post-race celebration cocktail. Those of us left were walking, or running very slowly, or some combination of both. My post-race celebration cocktail would have to wait, because I still had two miles to go.

That was one way to look at it. The other way to look at it was *I only had two miles to go.*

Three and a half hours ago I stood in front of the Rock & Roll Hall of Fame with 13.1 miles ahead of me and now I only had two miles left. Two miles. That's less than a 5K.

So I turned to the driver in the van, gave him a smile, and waved him off. Yes, I was okay. I was more than okay and there was no way in hell I was going to arrive at the finish line of my very first half marathon in a van.

And that's about the moment when I looked up ahead and saw my dad about a quarter mile away waiting for me. Knowing it was going to take me a couple of hours to complete the course, I had given my parents a rough estimate of when I expected to finish, and also had taken the additional step of signing my dad and sister up for the mobile tracking so they would be texted as I crossed certain mile markers. This meant that not only my sister, who lived 400 miles away in Alexandria, Virginia, would know the second I finished, but also my parents could keep an eye on my progress and know when to start heading downtown to meet me at the finish line.

I ran up ahead to greet my dad. As he gave me a high five, I asked how much further. (Actually, I'm pretty sure I asked, panting, "AM I CLOSE TO THE END?!") He waved ahead up Ontario Street and said it's just up and around the corner to the right, on Prospect Street.

A quarter mile. That was it. That was all that stood between me and the label Half-Marathoner. One single, solitary, small little quarter mile out of thirteen.

Thirteen is a heavy number. The fear of it is so strong that there is an entire phobia—triskaidekaphobia—built around it and woe if a Friday falls on that day during a normal calendar month. Things that come in sets of thirteen: The Original Colonies. A Baker's Dozen. The number of cards in a single suit of a standard deck.

Miles that I run? LOL.

Yet, here I was, the finish line literally around the corner. I took a deep breath and kept pushing myself. When my dad saw me pick up my pace, he picked up his own, too, and hurried up the street to take a short cut to beat me so he'd be there when I finished.

As I rounded the corner, I saw the big finish line sign hanging high above the city street. Because this particular Run Rock 'N' Roll race only had the half marathon, those of us finishing past the three hour mark were the very last of the bunch. By now, the crowd of spectators at the finish line had thinned out and they were starting to pack up some of the finisher's food and drink, knowing there were only a smattering of people still left on the course.

One of the spectators still waiting was my mom, who had managed to already snag me a bottle of water and a banana. She waved and snapped pictures as I hustled towards that finish line and crossed, finishing my very first half marathon in 3:37:53.

So I didn't meet my 3:30 goal but, really, it was okay. I may have been slow. I may have had to walk more than I would have liked. I may have even been so slow that there were faster runners capable of running twice that distance in the same amount of time.

But none of that mattered because *I had just become a half-marathoner*. I had joined a club that has only one entry requirement: complete a half marathon. Run, walk, whatever, just crush those 13.1 miles and membership is given.

At 311 pounds, I never in a million years would have ever conceived that I'd be able to call myself a runner, let alone a half-marathoner. And when the volunteer put the medal around my neck I couldn't stop smiling.

My goal had been to lose weight. In the end, I ended up finding myself.

9
It's a Major Award

In case it somehow isn't yet clear, I love Cleveland. And when I say I love Cleveland, what I really mean is that I FUCKING LOVE CLEVELAND.

Ask people what they know about the city of Cleveland and they'll probably say that our river once burned. Well, that and a certain basketball player. What they may not know is that Cleveland is a bit of a Midwest Hollywood, with several movies filmed here.

Next to my sheer adoration of Cleveland, I love watching movies. Along with major Hollywood blockbusters, Cleveland often plays host to a small smattering of independent films and I even have been an onscreen extra in one of them.

So, needless to say, my three favorite things are movies, races, and Cleveland. Not necessarily in that order because I pretty much love Cleveland more than I love anything else in the whole entire world. But, if you combine all three of my favorite loves, what do you get?

The Christmas Story 10K.

Oh yes, *A Christmas Story*. That annual holiday film that appears pretty much around the clock on Christmas Day about Ralphie and his Red Ryder Carbine Action 200-shot Range Model air rifle was filmed right here in good ol' Cleveland, Ohio. (Cue chorus of "You'll shoot your eye out, you'll shoot your eye out.") While the interior of the home where Ralphie lived with his mom, The Old Man, and his little brother Randy was located on a soundstage, the familiar exterior of the house is in the Tremont neighborhood. In the twenty-odd years since the film had been released, the home had gone through some cosmetic changes, including a new roof, new windows, and new siding. Driving past, it would have been hard for even the most devout fan to recognize the iconic home.

Then, in 2004, the owner put the house on eBay.

Because, really: when you are living in a filming location of a beloved holiday classic and want to sell it, where else would you post?

It was no surprise one of those devout fans bought the house. This was a fan that loves the film so much, he built a business around it, selling imitation leg lamps to other devout fans, complete with fishnet stockings and black high heels. He took the revenue from that small business to put a down payment on the house, buying it sight unseen off the internet. The house now stands as a museum.

My love for *A Christmas Story* is too numerous to name and like most Clevelanders, come December my halls are decked with leg lamps. (I actually have about a dozen all lined up together as a set of string lights.) Drive around the city during the holidays, and the Tremont neighborhood in particular, and the soft glow of electric sex gleams from window after window after window.

2013 marked the thirtieth anniversary of the iconic film and Cleveland was celebrating. One of the big events was a 10K. A 10K that I, kind of surprisingly, did *not* sign up for right away.

Here's the hard truth about themed novelty races: they tend to be more expensive than a usual 5K or 10K. Sometimes *significantly* more expensive. In Cleveland, a run-of-the-mill 5K averages about $25, a 10K maybe $30. The Christmas Story 5K/10K was $45 for early birds and $55 for everyone else.

I debated. I *agonized.* This was a race, in my city, themed around one of my absolute favorite movies. But ouch, that registration fee.

Then I saw a Groupon ad for 50 percent off and well, I do love me a good deal.

At the time of the inaugural Christmas Story 10K, I hadn't yet given into the fad of dressing up for races. Like dressing up, as in, y'know, costumes. It wasn't because I was worried about looking silly or anything: during the winter I often say (and many runners will back me up on this) that you know you're a runner when you don't care what you look like as long as you're warm.

I speak from personal experience on this one—I wear brightly colored running pants with whatever top I can find, sometimes layered with a long sleeve shirt underneath. Add a jacket and a set of earmuffs or a hat and who knows how ridiculous I appear to other people. But color coordination isn't exactly a priority—not freezing is all I care about.

That said, when I was planning my race day outfit for what was sure to be a very frigid race day, I realized I owned a pretty significant amount of pink athletic wear. Bright pink jacket. Bright pink knee high socks. Bright pink gloves. Hell, even my New Balance running shoes were a shade of neon pink so electric they practically glowed.

Everyone who has seen *A Christmas Story* knows that Ralphie, the main character, has an Aunt Clara who spent several years under the impression that Ralphie was not only four years old, but also a girl. Super awkward, especially when her gift to him one Christmas is a one-piece pink bunny costume. While Ralphie's mother finds the costume absolutely adorable, the Old Man (rightly) says the costume makes his son look like a pink nightmare.

Naturally, given the sheer amount of pink in my running wardrobe, I needed to represent that pink nightmare on race day.

And one of the benefits to having a mother who is a preschool teacher is being sure that there's a very good chance that she has a set of bunny ears available. A set of bunny ears that she'll be happy to let you borrow.

And thus, my first race day costume was born.

When planning the routes for the 5K and the 10K, the race committee opted to feature as many locations from *A Christmas Story* as possible. As it turns out, the *Christmas Story* house, which is located in the Tremont neighborhood, is three miles from downtown. Not just three miles from downtown, but three miles from Tower City Center which is home to the old Higbee's building.

In *A Christmas Story*, Higbee's was featured as the iconic storefront window from which Ralphie first spies his beloved BB gun and is also home to the department store where Ralphie goes to visit Santa Claus to ask for said gun. Santa, continuing the reaction shared by Ralphie's mother and teacher, tells Ralphie he'll shoot his eye out.

That these two locations are so close is magical—I can't even. It's as if the racing gods just knew that one day a race would be designed based on the film.

Or it could just be one big Hollywood coincidence called budgeting. But I'll let you be the judge.

I arrived at Tower City Center with lots of time to spare, mostly owing to the fact that I had no idea what the parking situation would be like and always a Type A, I wanted to give myself plenty of wiggle room. The indoor shopping center was bursting with runners, most in costumes familiar to even a casual fan. We crowded together in the atrium near Public Square because ZOMG IT WAS SO FUCKING COLD. BODY HEAT PLEASE.

I suddenly envied those runners who had chosen to dress in the adult-sized version of the pink bunny pajamas that the museum sold in their gift shop. Those were some damn smart runners, let me tell you.

With maybe twenty minutes until the gun went off, all that coffee I had consumed prior to leaving the house was starting to catch up with my bladder. Unfortunately, it seemed like everyone else's bladders were feeling the same way because the lines outside of the shopping center's public restrooms were crazy long. Even that one restroom off to the side, all the way down that one corridor that almost no one knew existed had been discovered.

Then it occurred to me that I could just pop into the Horseshoe Casino and use their restrooms . . . only about a half a second later, it also occurred to me that in my attempt to pack light, I had left my driver's license at home, so I had no way to verify I was old enough to even enter the casino.

My only option was to just suck it up, and hope I could make it through the race without having to stop and use a porta-potty.

With a few minutes left on the clock, all of the runners started the mass exodus out of Tower City and into the streets surrounding Public Square. A large film screen had been set up on one of the sidewalks and was showing the film on a loop while we waited.

Unfortunately, because we were all crowded into such a small area, it created a bottleneck when the race officially started. Tucked in the back as usual, it took a lot longer to get up to the start line than I had anticipated, and there were lots of faster runners dispersed in the back because there was no easy way for them to get up front where they belonged.

It was, in some ways, a bit of a clusterfuck.

Eventually, though, it was my turn and my race started. The course turned left onto Ontario Street, one of the major roads in the city. We passed the Quicken Loans Arena, home of the Cleveland Cavaliers, and Progressive Field, home of the Cleveland Indians, before turning right onto the Lorain-Carnegie Bridge.

Of course, despite how many times I've driven across the bridge, I always forget how long it is. Just months before, I'd run across the bridge for the Run Rock 'N' Roll Half Marathon and yet I somehow had forgotten that it's a beast of a bridge, over a mile entirely on its own.

At the other end of the bridge, the course turned left onto Abbey Road. Sadly, no Beatles were in sight. But we ran along Abbey Road another mile or so to West 11th Street.

This is the same street all my friends live on—the same friends who were out with signs and cheers back in October during my half marathon. But for some reason, they weren't out at 8 a.m. on a cold, chilly December morning. Gosh. How shocking.

For those of us running the 10K, this marked about two miles into the race, or a little less than a third of the way done; on the other hand, the 5K runners were nearly finished, those lucky bastards. The snow had started to fall—thick, heavy, huge white flakes that stuck to my pink jacket instead of melting away.

Now the race committee definitely had fun planning this race. Along the course were white A-frame posts that included bits of film trivia, like the fact that Jack Nicholson had been sent a script of the film for the role of the father. (That would have made for a *very* different film, amirite?)

Being that this was an out-and-back course, as I ran along 11th Street towards the house, the faster 10K runners were running along 11th Street in the opposite direction. From my vantage point, I was able to see lots of really clever costumes. My favorite was a woman with red hair wearing a dress similar to that of Ralphie's mom *carrying a turkey on a tray*. Like, with both hands. That takes a special level of dedication. It's one thing to run carrying, say, a phone or iPod in your hand. Then a runner can still pump his or her arms while he or she runs like a normal person. With this bird, the runner's hands had to be outstretched in front of her, and not only were they outstretched in front of her but she had to use them to carry something for the entire 6.2 miles. Did she have to practice this before? Train while carrying the tray? SO. MANY. QUESTIONS.

Right around the Mile Three mark, the course turned from 11th onto Rowley Avenue. The *Christmas Story* House and Museum is tucked way back in this little neighborhood. It's really the last place a person would expect to find a museum, which, I mean, makes sense when you consider that part of the house's appeal to the filmmakers probably was the fact that it is tucked away in a little neighborhood. In fact, the first time I went looking for it years ago, I almost nearly drove right past it because I think I was just looking for something a little bit more . . . well, fancy. I mean, HELLO. This is the house from *A CHRISTMAS STORY*. How are there not many big signs and flashing lights and a red carpet? THIS SHOULD BE A MAJOR TOURIST DESTINATION FOR FILM LOVERS EVERYWHERE.

Turning the corner, I spotted the finish line for the 5K up ahead. The house was a backdrop to a balloon arch and finish line. A crowd of spectators had gathered around to cheer on the 5K finishers.

After snapping a quick picture of the festive house with my phone, I turned and continued on my way. The house was only my halfway point.

There was a small loop around the neighborhood that put me back on 11th Street. Being a slow runner, the view from this side of the street and course was different. There was no line of runners on the other side of the street heading towards the house; it was simply those of us in the back of the pack heading downtown.

Around Mile Five, I succumbed to the curse of runners everywhere— my bladder started to catch up with me. I had a mile to go, but that was almost all going to be on and over the Hope Memorial (aka the Lorain-Carnegie) Bridge. If I didn't stop at the row of porta-potties on this side of the bridge, I wouldn't have another opportunity to stop.

I weighed my ability to hold it for another mile and change against how distracting and uncomfortable it would be to hold it in for another mile. I decided to stop.

Stepping out of the porta-potty when I was done, I set my sights on the final stretch of the race: up and over the Hope Memorial Bridge, then down Ontario for a stretch, before turning back towards Public Square and the finish line.

The snow was falling pretty heavily by now and the fat flakes were sticking to the ground. The bunny ears were proving to be a less than stellar choice on my part, as they worked against the wind rather than with it. After having to adjust them more than once, I ended up taking the bunny ears off and tucking them into the pink jacket until the end of the race.

The back of the pack had thinned out considerably by now, and I'd been alone for a while, the only runner in sight. As I turned that final corner and looked up ahead towards the finish line, I saw my parents waiting up ahead for me. I reached into my pink jacket and pulled out the bunny ears. Planting them firmly on my head, I just hoped they'd stay in place long enough for me to finish.

Crossing the finish line, I breathed a cold sigh of relief. It was freezing and snowy and I hadn't run my best, finishing well over an hour and a half. That porta-potty stop didn't help and the cold surely slowed me down some.

The volunteer handed me my finisher's medal, which proudly displays the iconic *A Christmas Story* leg lamp in a running position with a large wooden box marked FRAGILE on it. On the bottom it was written IT'S A MAJOR AWARD.

As I posed for a picture with my dad in front of the famous Higbee's building, the medal hanging around my neck, I remembered there is more to running and racing than time. Sometimes there is a really cool fucking medal, too.

10

The Longest Four Miles of My Life

As I slowly pulled my shoe off my right foot I grimaced. There was sharp pain stabbing my heel and once I extracted my foot from my shoe, the first thing I noticed was a bright red spot of blood on the back of my sock.

Fuck.

It was mid-May 2014 and I was a week away from my second half marathon and had just completed ten miles, the longest long run of my training plan. Anticipating that the ten miles was going to take me a while, I had gotten to Edgewater Park by 6:30 that morning. From my vantage point on the top of the hill, I was able to watch the sun rise over the Cleveland skyline three miles away.

With this final long run completed, my tapering phase was about to, thankfully, begin.

As all smart runners know, there are a few universal rules when racing: one is don't ever wear anything new on race day. Those fabulous new shoes bought on sale at the expo? Keep them in the box until *after* your half marathon. That free shirt that came with the packet? Save it for later: it's the perfect way to brag about the race just completed at a post-race brunch. Also, I know the capris or shorts you just had to have make your lower half look awesome, but keep them packed away for just a few more days.

The downside to this is that if you're me, and find that my running shoes all of a sudden hate me a few days before your big race, I'm kind of out of luck. I'd been wearing the same style of shoe for several years now, just buying a new pair every few months or so, and I'd never had this problem before where the back of the shoe was rubbing up against my heel and ankle. Being so close to race day, this was not the time to change horses—or shoes, as it were—midstream. The alternative was to buy a new pair of the same style, and just hope that I happened to have a faulty pair, but even then, because I was tapering, I didn't know if I'd have enough time to both break them in while also giving my body the much needed break it required after so many months of training. I was kind of screwed.

The thing is, three months ago, the Cleveland Half Marathon wasn't even on my radar, but when someone provides you with a free race entry you shouldn't let it go to waste.

Like many race organizations, the Cleveland Marathon takes advantage of social media–savvy runners by naming them Ambassadors. In exchange for a comped entry and fun swag, these racing Ambassadors chronicle training and race progress on their blogs, thus encouraging other runners to register. Some races only give the free entry if and when an Ambassador drums up enough registrations, but Cleveland gives it as part of the package. Ambassadors also are provided with an additional free entry that they can give away on their blog, which is how I found myself with one such Golden Ticket in February 2014.

A year ago, in the spring of 2013, I followed up my successful ConocoPhillips 10K with the Cleveland 10K, one of the many distances offered by the Cleveland Marathon organization. I had briefly considered running the 10K again but races are expensive yo, and I was trying to be a boring fiscally responsible adult. (Sigh.)

Once I realized I could possibly win an entry, I was all over that shit, entering every single giveaway as they cropped up across the local blogosphere. Because of the sheer size of the Cleveland running community, entries into each giveaway are pretty substantial, always making winning a long shot, but I got lucky and ended up winning a race entry.

When I was notified of my very own Golden Ticket at the end of February, my gut reaction was to register for the 10K like I had planned. But then when I sat down and looked at my calendar, I realized that if I started training right away, as in the following Monday, I'd be right on schedule to rock my second half marathon.

A second half wasn't on my agenda. Like, at all. Especially not six months after my first. Hell, when I crossed that finish line back in October, I was so happy just to have finished a half marathon, I didn't give any thought to ever running another one. But here I was, with a free entry handed to me exactly twelve weeks before the race. Given the circumstances, how could I *not* plan on running the half marathon?

So here I was, twelve weeks later. The countdown to the 2014 Cleveland Half Marathon was in the single digits and my shoes were causing my feet to bleed.

As I've said, racing rituals come with all experienced runners. Me, I like to carefully set everything out on my dining room table the night before: shirt, pants, shoes, socks, bib, pins, earbuds, running belt and/ or armband, charged phone, and fuel if I'm running a longer distance race. This way, when I wake up, I know that everything I need for race day is already sitting there waiting and I won't have to start searching through my closet at 6 a.m., still blurry from sleep.

I also like to get a manicure the day before, then go home that night and work on my running playlist while drinking wine.

(YOU DO YOU, OKAY?)

Normally I just use my regular "workout" playlist, set that puppy on random, and I'm good to go. But this time I was taking a slightly different approach. For the first time, I was experimenting with walking intervals and I wanted to use the music as an auditory cue for when I needed to change my pace.

The idea of walking initially came from a spin class where we have moments of "active recovery," a less intense workout that comes in the middle of a longer workout. So it's not a full-on rest, but it does give the body a small break while still working it, hence the *active* part. Adding in walking breaks to my half marathon plan was a great way to get those periods of active recovery and my plan was 12 to 13 minutes of running followed by 3 minutes of walking.

(I have *zero* idea where I came up with those numbers, since, well, math; they really just kind of sounded good.)

At the suggestion of a friend, I decided to take advantage of Spotify's impressive collection of military cadences to signal when it was time to walk. The "I don't know but I've been told" sort of thing. In order for this work, I had to actually put together a playlist in a somewhat specific order. Because this was based on time, I needed to match songs up in a way they filled that roughly 12- to 13-minute timeframe, without going over too far.

Again, this meant doing math. While drinking.

Yeah, really well thought-out plan there, Jill.

Once my playlist was complete and my glass of wine polished off, I crawled into bed for an early night. With all the necessary road closures, I was going to have to be parked downtown and headed towards my corral well before sunrise.

I don't know if it was excitement, nerves, or what, but I was wide awake at 4:30 a.m. I tried going back to sleep for another hour or so, but it soon became clear that wasn't going to happen, so I got out of bed and got dressed. Sitting on the edge of my bed, I examined my feet.

The backs of my ankles were still red and raw and I knew that as soon as I put those shoes back on they were going to get rubbed even more, exasperating the wounds. Using some of the *Monsters, Inc.* bandages in my bathroom (I make zero apologies for my love of Pixar as a thirtysomething), I covered those wounds as best I could. The packet I had picked up at the Convention Center the day before also included some clear bandage-type strips and I put those on top of Mike and Sully.

(I had Boo over my boo-boo. #Sorrynotsorry.)

With my ankles covered as sufficiently as I was going to manage this particular morning, I decided I might as well gather my gear and head over towards the start. If nothing else, I was at least going to get a decent parking spot.

They were still setting up the start line when I arrived. I found a spot to hang out while I watched them erect the START banner and lay the blue mats underneath. This was a new experience: as a slow runner I have, unfortunately, been witness to them tearing the course *down* but I'd never seen them put it up.

Standing on the corner of Superior Avenue, the crest of Terminal Tower rising high, with the sunrise peeking over the city skyline, I could sense my right foot was going to be an issue. It wasn't really hurting and I could still walk and everything, but something felt . . . off. This new discomfort, combined with the back of my ankles, was suddenly making me regret opting to run the half marathon over the 10K. Too late now.

Having done the training, the last thing I wanted to do was just quit, but I wasn't aware I had another option, which was run the 10K anyway. At the 2016 races, there was snow and hail. In mid-May. If that's not the most Cleveland race ever, I don't know what else is. Because of the drastic change in weather, several runners ended up switching to one of the shorter distances at one of the course splits. Back then, it didn't occur to me as something I could do. I thought it was Run the Half Marathon or Don't Run the Half Marathon.

So, I chose to run the half marathon, fucked-up feet and all.

At 7 a.m., the race organizers started releasing the corrals. I was in the last corral, the one with the walkers, which meant there was the usual lag time between the start of the race and when I actually got up to the line. My right foot was still bugging me, but I forged ahead. Pulling my phone out of my belt, I brought up Spotify and pressed the Play button on my new running playlist as soon as I crossed the start line.

We started downtown at Public Square, which was a new start for me, but a nice change as I usually don't get to run right downtown thanks to, y'know, cars and buses and stuff. After winding our way in and around the streets for a couple of miles, we headed across the Hope Memorial Bridge.

Halfway across the bridge, the watchful eyes of the Guardians of Traffic loomed. These tall statues represent various modes of transportation and safely guard those crossing the bridge. It was here that the race courses diverged. Everything was color-coded: green for the 10K, red for the half marathon, and blue for the full marathon. Bibs matched the color and the runners were instructed to follow the color-coded signs along the course.

In the very middle of the bridge, right around the Mile Three mark, there was a yellow sandwich board with colored boxes and arrows. The 10K runners went off toward the right side of the bridge and the half and full marathon runners stuck to the left side. At the other end of the bridge, we turned in different directions and went our separate ways.

Now, earlier in the week I had signed up my dad and sister for the real-time mobile tracking. Everyone knew I was running this race, including my entire social media feed, which I had also signed up for real-time tracking. I even signed *myself* up for the real-time tracking—checking my phone for the automatic text every time I crossed one of the blue mats along the course was going to be the best way to monitor my pace.

For the half marathon, this meant that when I hit the 10K mat, also known as the halfway point, I was able to pull my phone out a few seconds later to read the automated text that came through.

My average pace at the halfway point was 17:24 per mile, which put me almost a minute per mile behind my pace from October's Run Rock 'N' Roll Half Marathon, but my foot *was* bothering me so I forgave my speed a little more than I perhaps normally would have.

The next two miles went by, I was keeping up my intervals of 12 to 13 minutes of running followed by 3 minutes of walking. Rinse and repeat. Along the way, the half marathon and the full marathon courses split—I was only a few miles away from the finish while the full marathoners had a good ten, at least, to go.

Around Mile Eight, my right foot started to act up. Not a scream, not quite yet. This was more like a whimper. A light dull throb that quietly, but insistently, made its presence known with each step I took.

I fought and forced my way through the next mile, but as soon as I hit that marker for Mile Nine, I knew there was no physical way for me to run any further so I switched to walking.

The Cleveland Marathon races all start downtown. The exact location of the start line has shifted and changed over the years, from behind First Merit Stadium, to Public Square, to in front of First Merit Stadium, but the *end* is always on Lakeside Avenue. All the distances start and end together. There may be some separation between the two, as each runs the full length of each course, but eventually they all merge together onto the Cleveland Memorial Shoreway.

Connecting the East and West Sides of the city, the Shoreway is a freeway that runs parallel to the coast of Lake Erie. Rising high above the city, from my vantage point in the final stretch of the race I was able to see my apartment building far below.

My apartment, which sits along the banks of the mighty Cuyahoga River. It was so fucking hot out, I kept glancing over the barrier and thinking *man that water looks nice and cool.*

Yup, I was so hot I was contemplating the logistics of swimming in a river that once caught on fire.

The course for the Cleveland Half Marathon has changed slightly since, but in 2014, the final four miles of the race was entirely on the Shoreway. These final four miles are four miles on hard concrete, the sun mercilessly beating down. That high up, there's no coverage from trees or awnings and this was one of those blistering days in the middle of May when the sun is just so happy to finally be free from the cold chains of winter that it's just flashing everybody.

Along with signing myself up for the automatic updates along the course, I also set it up so that those same updates would be posted to my Facebook page. Because that's what we do these days: it's simply not enough to post a finish time a few minutes after the race has ended, once the post-finish chocolate milk and banana have been consumed. Oh no, these have to be posted so fast that unless I'm holding my phone in my hand and look down at the screen as soon as I finish—my entire social media following is going to know how I did before I do.

The thing is, those automatic updates being posted on my behalf only work well when my body is working well. Otherwise I'm just that girl hobbling along the freeway frantically typing a Facebook post as I slowly walk explaining that my finish time is going to be nowhere near the time stupid auto post indicated seven miles ago.

Obviously posting on social media would be a low priority for most people in the middle of a half marathon. Only, I knew people were watching and waiting and I knew that when I crossed that finish line and that ridiculous tracker posted to my Facebook page, it would give a finishing time of over four hours. Really, I was just trying to do damage control and make sure to explain *why* I'd be finishing so slowly.

Plus, I mean, hi, I was walking. Slowly. Might as well update Facebook and Twitter and maybe scroll through my Instagram photo feed while I was at it. Anything to distract from the reality of my situation at that moment in time.

Look, I am completely OK with my speed, okay? I'm totally fine being slow and making jokes about being a turtle and blah blah blah. But personally, for me, an over four hour half marathon was about the limit of my self-acceptance on the slow runner front. I don't say this as a means of disparaging runners slower than I am—speed, like so much else about running, is a very personal thing and everyone has their own thresholds of comfort when it comes to identifying paces we are okay with running. For me, this was well outside my comfort zone of being okay.

I physically felt horrible and I mentally and emotionally felt horrible and I was so over it. I was over the whole thing. This stupid race. This stupid running. This stupid heat and these really, really stupid four miles that had officially become the bane of my very existence. My feet were fucking killing me, I was sweating buckets, and I probably had a sunburn. All I wanted to do was sit down on the side of the Shoreway and cry and wait for some kind soul in an air-conditioned car to come pick me up.

Bonus points if they had magically known to pick up a pint of local Mitchell's Ice Cream Campfire S'mores flavor. (Technically, that particular seasonal variety doesn't come out until later in the summer, hence why they'd need to be *magical*.)

But, of course, there was no air-conditioned car and there was no roasted marshmallow ice cream with chocolate chunks and homemade graham cracker pieces.

There was just me. Limping along the longest four fucking miles of my entire fucking life.

I was officially fucking done with this entire fucking thing.

But, see, the thing is, the only thing I hated more than those four miles was the idea of leaving this race unfinished. A DNF—a Did Not Finish—was not a part of my half marathon training plan and with less than a mile to go there was no way in hell I was actually going to quit now.

Hobbling my way down the exit ramp, I spotted my cousin Michele and her daughter Katy waiting for me. As soon as Michele saw me, she jumped off the barrier she'd been using as a chair and started leaping into the air, cheering, with her arms raised high above her. With every jump, she'd spread her legs out and do big ol' circles with her arms. As if she was afraid I somehow wouldn't see her otherwise.

Which, granted, she's incredibly petite, but I had no idea she could be so *loud* for having such a tiny body.

(Vocal volume is a bit of a family trait, not gonna lie.)

It was, admittedly, a bit mortifying. (LOVE YOU, MICHELE!) This particular half marathon was going to take me over four hours to complete and by that time there was almost nobody left on the half marathon course. All the other spectators were there for the full marathon runners. The respectability of finishing a half marathon in four hours versus a full marathon in 4 hours is vastly different. A 4-hour marathon is damn impressive. A 4-hour half marathon, not so much.

How dare I call myself a runner.

Then there's my cousin, a pretty decent runner herself, with multiple marathons behind her, completely unable to contain her excitement at getting to see me cross the finish line.

I was so exhausted and so ready to just be fucking *done* with this whole stupid thing, it hadn't really sunk it quite yet what I was about to do, which was complete my second half marathon.

With both Michele and Katy now cheering for me, I picked up my pace as fast as my poor feet would allow. I'd like to say I ran. I didn't. Nor would I even use the dreaded "J" word and say I jogged. This was more of a . . . shuffle.

But shuffle I did. One foot in front of the other, slowly (oh so slowly) but surely. It hurt and those bandages I so carefully put on that morning where all rubbed off by the time I got home, but step by step I made it to that finish line and I crossed it.

In the end, I completed my second half marathon with an average pace of 19 minutes and 17 seconds. It took me 4 hours, 12 minutes, and 38 seconds to finish those 13.1 miles.

But I fucking finished.

11
Will Run For Bling

Signing up for an 8 a.m. race on November 1 sounded good in theory, up until that panicked moment when I realized that it meant Halloween, my absolute favorite holiday ever, was not only the night before, but was also a rare year where the actual holiday lines up with a weekend.

When it comes to Halloween, I tend to go a bit extreme. Exhibit A: my birthday is in mid-November and one year during high school I decided I didn't want a birthday party but, instead, wanted a Halloween party. At sixteen, I had recently discovered the magic and mayhem that is *The Rocky Horror Picture Show* and not only did I dress up as the domestic Magenta, but at my Halloween party I made all of my friends dance the Time Warp. (As it happens, they were all more than happy to oblige, which explains why we are still all friends to this day.)

For me, Halloween is a serious endeavor: costumes are planned and worked on months in advance. I also have *feelings* when it comes to celebrating on any day beyond October 31, which means years when Halloween falls on a Thursday are challenging. Do I dress up and choose to paint the town black and orange a full week before? Or do I go for the weekend closest to the holiday, even if means celebrating in November?

The last day of October in 2014 was a Friday and my friends and I—All Hallows Eve aficionados all—had been strategizing our group costume since early summer. Because, for us, Halloween is not just an evening to stick some cheap devil horns on your head and throw on a red dress and call it a night. Halloween is an *event* for us.

We had plans, you see. Big plans with big costumes. Costumes that involved papier-mâché and do-it-yourself and illusions. Plans and costumes that did not work well with an 8 a.m. 5K the next morning.

My decision to register for the Bernie Kosar 5K came on the heels of the Rock 'N' Roll Marathon series decision to cancel the 2014 Cleveland races. Which came on the heels of my completely and utterly losing my running mojo.

My second half marathon back in May did *not* go well. Like, at all. The thing was, that wasn't even supposed to be my second half marathon but then I won the entry and, well, I can totally run two half marathons in a single year, right?

I ran the Cleveland Half in May but after that experience pretty much wanted to quit running altogether. But then I won another free entry to a race a couple weeks later, this time the Copper River Salmon 5K. I went in with zero expectations, didn't worry about time or pace and it ended up being just what I needed to make up for the Cleveland Half.

Then July came and I needed to start training for the Run Rock 'N' Roll Half. In the beginning, I was all for it—this would be my comeback story! Redemption Road Racing! It was going to be great.

Except it wasn't. The training was horrible. I felt horrible. I had to force myself to complete every single workout; it was just awful. So then, about a month into my training I decided to drop from the half marathon to the 10K.

So when, in early September 2014, about one month before race day, when the RnR organization full on cancelled the *entire* Cleveland races, I was more than a little upset. Had I still been planning on running the half marathon I would no doubt have been relieved by this change in situation, but I was looking forward to the 10K. Now I had nothing to look forward to. I felt like all that training was for naught.

Because it's such a big organization, with lots of "tour stops" along the way, transfers were allowed. They even connected with the main

Rite Aid Cleveland Marathon organization and allowed transfers into one of those races.

But, they also gave refunds. Which is how I ended up with enough extra moola to justify signing up for the Bernie Shuffle 5K, so named in honor of one of Cleveland's more memorable NFL figures.

Sports? Not really my thing. Of course, I also live in Cleveland. Sports in this city are fraught with tension. Titles not won, game after game, the mantra of *There's always next year* echoing throughout each stadium at the end of another season. There was always next year, fifty-two years' worth of next years, and while LeBron & Co. brought the championship home in 2016, at the time of the Bernie Shuffle 5K, we were still several years away from breaking the Cleveland Curse.

It wasn't all bad. We've had our moments. The Indians back in the 1990s and the Cavs, of course. The Browns, however . . .

There have been a small handful of men to come out of their time in the Browns camp as local heroes. The one whose legacy has lasted the longest is Bernie Kosar, who played for the Browns from 1985 until 1993. It was this Bernie that was the namesake for the Bernie Shuffle, a 5K to be held on November 1, 2014. Which, again, made sense at that time. Up until I looked at my calendar, that is.

(Course maps. Calendars. I really have to work on those.)

Novelty races often come with hefty swag, which in turn creates a hefty registration fee. Usually I am not one to fork over $45 for a mere 5K, especially one that is considered a "fun run" and untimed. But in the case of the Bernie Kosar 5K I could not get over the Herculean, super sparkly, super shiny finisher's medal. When this race was first announced I found myself staring in awe at the medal but, at the time, could not make my bank account work with it.

Now, though, money in hand, I wanted that medallion. I *coveted* that medallion. I HAD TO HAVE THAT MEDALLION. That super sparkly, super shiny behemoth needed to join the other medals hanging from the rack in my living room. It would be the center, my showcase piece.

But I also wanted to go out on Halloween and enjoy myself and flaunt the obscene amount of man-hours that went into my costume without worrying about getting home early enough to be rested for a 5K the next morning.

All week I waffled, knowing my decision to run would be a game day decision. Which seemed fitting, considering this was a race theme based on an NFL sports franchise.

On Friday, October 31, I went out with my friends as Halloween-ified as I could get. Despite the weekend date on the calendar, not many people were out in their costumes, so we tended to be the freak group of folks at the bar dressed up. (And I mean "freak" literally—our group costume for the year was sideshow carnival acts. I was the legless woman, being carried around by my assistant. I gave him a name and everything. Like I said, we take Halloween very, very seriously.)

As we climbed into bed at 2:30 a.m., still drunk from that evening's festivities, I told my boyfriend it was decided: I was going to run the Bernie Shuffle 5K and promptly set my alarm.

When said alarm clock went off four hours later, I woke with a groan, head smarting with the start of a small hangover. Because, of course, that's what happens when you drink too much and go to sleep really late. I'm also old. Not, like, really old but over the past few years I had discovered that thirtysomething Jill cannot hold her liquor quite the same way as twentysomething Jill could. Also, while I easily pulled all-nighters in college, nowadays anything less than seven hours of sleep made for a very, very cranky Jill in the morning.

Then I made the mistake of looking outside.

It was *snowing*.

I really started to question last night's game day decision.

Honestly, this is the reason big life decisions should not be made after a person has consumed copious amounts of alcohol while celebrating her favorite holiday.

There was, quite literally, only one thing stopping me from crawling back into bed and burrowing myself under the covers:

The stupid fucking medal. That stupid, fucking, really cool, and really beautiful medal.

As much as I coveted that damn thing, I was starting to loathe it. Oh sure it's all big and sparkly and fabulous but if it wasn't for that stupid sparkly fabulous thing I could remain in the cozy confines of my bed. Instead, I was trying to figure out the best way to both stay warm and show off my costume. Because, I mean, if you're going to run a race the day after Halloween you might as well dress up? Because, really, why else would you have a race then? Granted, my 2014 Halloween costume was a little bit too complicated for race wear so I was instead repurposing my 2013 Halloween costume, which was the TARDIS. From *Doctor Who*. Because I am a geek. And I keep a suitcase full of all previous costumes. Because you just never know when a costume may be needed.

So I had on my blue shirt with a second long sleeve blue shirt underneath and a pair of black yoga pants and TARDIS knee-high socks and a blue bow in my hair because bow ties are cool. Just a few months before, at the Cleveland Flea, a big outdoor arts, crafts, and vintage event in the city, I had purchased a set of fingerless crocheted gloves styled after the costume of choice for Matt Smith's Eleventh Doctor, so I slipped those over my hands and hopped in the car.

The Bernie Shuffle 5K started at Voinovich Park, a small manmade park on the harbor of Lake Erie. The Rock & Roll Hall of Fame and Museum acts as a backdrop to the park, which features neat landscaping and a small stage that is utilized in the summer.

Because the park is basically at the dead end of a pier, it's not the most convenient location in the city, but it wasn't the getting to the race part I was concerned about: it was the getting home *after* the race part. There is parking down in that area, but I had a feeling that trying to leave after I was done was going to be a hot mess, so I opted to park a couple blocks away and walk to the starting line.

It was dark. It was cold. It was snowy and hailing and just about whatever kind of precipitation exists was probably falling from the sky. Aside from two races the month before, I had done almost zero running since May. Oh yeah, I also came in last place in one of them, and really wasn't looking forward to a repeat performance of that. After six months of just no good, horrible running, I needed *something* positive to keep me going. I needed to recapture that running magic that convinced me to step on that treadmill for the first time two and a half years ago.

As I walked down the hill towards Voinovich Park, I decided I was just going to walk the entire thing.

It was a fun run, which meant it was untimed. So, it's not like anyone was going to know how I did anyway unless I took the initiative to time myself, but this was also my last race of the year and coming off a previous last place finish I just wanted a stress-free morning. I wanted to start and I wanted to finish and if the only way that was going to happen was if I walked, then walking it would be.

As the race began, all the participants stood in a big crowd in Voinovich Park, trying to stay warm. The close proximity to Lake Erie was so not helping in that regard. Lake-effect snow? It's a thing. Precipitation brought on by large bodies of water? Also a thing. And there we were, standing right by a large body of water, freezing our asses off. Of course, some of the runners who were clearly smarter than I was had decided to wear their Browns gear, which meant sweatshirts and hoodies, while I decided to be clever and wear a fucking Halloween costume barely warm enough for fall, let alone winter.

As the runners around me were bouncing up and down in place to generate some heat, I was on my phone, fiddling around with the music player to queue up my workout songs. I decided that even if the race organization behind the Bernie Shuffle wasn't going to have any sort of official timing mechanism in place, I at least wanted to know how I did, in addition to starting up my Spotify app, I also opened up the clock app on my phone. Since I was running a predetermined distance, I only needed to know how long it took me to finish, so I didn't have any need for one of my fancier apps that would also track mileage. The really basic stopwatch application on the phone would do just fine.

As I waited, I looked around, surprised at how many people had shown up for the race. I discovered on that very cold, very overcast morning, even with the hefty registration fees, that those who really love the theme will brave the cold and the snow for that sweet, sweet swag. Even with the horrendous weather, there was quite a large turnout for the race and, following the usual slow runner and walker protocol, I tucked myself into a spot in the back.

The race started and the crowd surged forward up the brick pier towards downtown.

I walked a couple of yards then looked to my left, where a small crowd of people were gathered. Everyone was excited and I saw multiple phones raised high, snapping pictures.

Curious, I went over to see what all the fuss was about.

Oh. My. God. It was Bernie Kosar.

There, in the flesh, was the man whose name graced the race we were currently all running. Even for a non-sports (and definitely a non-football) fan like myself, it was a pretty cool experience to see him, right there on the course. I snapped a quick photo then kept on walking.

These were not runners who were also Browns fans. These were Browns fans first. Browns fans who decided, *Hey, I'm gonna go do this race because it's Bernie Kosar themed.* Browns fans who, for the most part, weren't runners at all. Not even a little bit, like not even close. The back of the pack was huge and comprised of mostly walkers, proudly sporting their orange and brown jerseys.

For once, I found myself in something more akin to the *middle* of the pack.

Because I wasn't worried about my pace or time, the normal stress that comes with chasing the finish line of the past few months vanished and I was really just able to enjoy myself. It had been months since I'd felt so free and even fast, despite the fact that I was walking the whole thing. It was snowing and cold and I should have been miserable, but I was having a blast.

I had never really before noticed how lonely I tended to feel during races, too. Most of the races I run don't have quite so many people and even those that are large tend to thin out soon after the race starts and I'm left in the back almost all alone. Oh sure, there are other runners back there with me, but our paces are all a little haphazard, so that we aren't keeping up with each other or trying to maintain the same pace like in the front and middle of the pack. I'm usually running all alone with runners a few yards ahead or behind me, but never with them on either side.

In that way, being in the back of the pack is kind of like being an elite runner.

With this, though, I was surrounded. It was fantastic and a very different experience that probably added to my good mood. Instead of feeling like a pressure-filled race, it was like taking a long walk with 1,000 of my not-so-closest friends.

Of course, they were all wearing orange and brown and I stuck out like a sore TARDIS in my bright blue BUT WHATEVER. If Doctor Who just magically landed in Cleveland on that particular day, he'd easily be able to find me, which is all that mattered.

As I crossed the finish line, I pulled out my phone to pause the stopwatch app that had been running the whole time I was walking. 57 minutes and 18 seconds. That means I walked an 18 minute and 29 second mile over the course of three miles. I was okay with that.

Up ahead, at the end of the pier, a pair of women were handing out the finisher's medals. Grinning, I bent forward as one of the women put the medal around my neck.

It was even more gorgeous in person.

The ribbon was a bright orange with thin strips of brown and white running down the sides. In the center hung the biggest, most sparkly, most fabulous racing medal I have ever seen. Silver crystals sparkled on the rim, with the words BERNIE SHUFFLE and 2014 etched in metal. The orange center glittered against the sun, the big brown B in the very middle outshining them all.

To think I almost sacrificed this beautiful behemoth for something as silly as *sleep*.

I mean, really.

Medal hanging proudly around my neck, I walked the quarter of a mile or so back to my car and turned the heat on as high as it would go. Once home, I took a shower that just about used up all the hot water, then climbed back into bed for a nap.

After waking up, I took my medal and hung it smack dab in the middle of my medal rack. That huge sparkly B outranked all of my other medals, and as I put it in its proper place, they all jostled slightly, the clinking and clanking of medal against medal music to my ears.

Not all runs, not all races, are going to be awesome. Some are just going to fucking suck and as a slow runner, the odds are in my favor that I'll come in last place every once in a while. Sometimes the body needs a reset. Sometimes the mind does, too. Sometimes that means waking up early and walking an entire 5K while cold and tired (and, admittedly, slightly hung over).

It's worth it, though. Because as I took a step back and gazed at my new medal, nestled among my other medals, I was able to calculate all the miles I had run to earn those finisher's medals and additionally, I was able to calculate all the training miles that got me to all of those finish lines.

Step by step, mile by mile. These were my medals and I had worked hard for each and every single one of them and no matter what happened, no matter how horrible I may have felt on race day, those medals represent the blood, sweat, and tears that went into making me the runner I am today.

Not everyone approves of finisher's medals. They liken them to the participation trophies that overwhelm elementary school sports across the country. The only people who deserve medals, the logic goes, are those runners fast enough to win their age groups.

The thing is, the back of the pack deserves medals, too. We are out there for longer, putting in just as much work and energy. We run alone for miles at a time. We love the sport as much as the faster runners ahead of us. Yes, sometimes we come in last place and, yes, this is a race. But our miles count just as much even if we don't run them as fast.

When it comes to last place, it's really sometimes luck of the draw. Sometimes I'm the slowest person who shows up for a race and I get that police escort all to myself. Other times, slower runners brave the long and lonely miles.

It goes both ways, too. When a fast runner places in their age group, it's because they happened to be one of the fastest runners who showed up that day. But another day, another race, another faster runner could show up and bump them from the top spot.

Those miles were still completed, the race still finished. Which is why I love finisher's medals so much. Because, unlike a faster runner, I don't have the chance of possibly placing in my age group. So having a medal to hang and visually represent all of the races I've run reminds me on a daily basis that yes, I'm slow. Yes, I've come in last place before and probably will again. But I'm still a *runner*, no matter what.

I run and run and run, and I have the bling to prove it.

12
Forward Is a Pace

This is the story of a loser.

That word, *loser*. It is a complex, multilayered word. We can lose jobs, lose lovers, and even lose ourselves for a bit.

But it's not always bad, losing things. We can also lose weight. Sometimes, with hard work and dedication, it can be a significant amount of weight.

But like a set of keys misplaced and lost in an apartment, these things can be found.

Or, in the case of lost weight, these things can be regained.

I started 2013 weighing roughly 175 pounds and running just under a 14-minute mile. Then, well. Life happened. The shit, as it were, hit the proverbial fan and I took it all in the face. Drama. Oh, the drama. Job drama. Boy drama. So much drama I could have gotten on stage and won a fucking Tony for the amount of drama in my life at that time.

So, I did what any fat girl with food issues and low self-esteem does: I started to eat.

I was still running consistently and in the fall of that year I had completed my first half marathon. Of course, training for a half marathon gave me the mental excuse to overeat because, *hello*, I was training.

Proper running nutrition still eludes me slightly to this day, but it really eluded me in the beginning. I heard "carbo load" and interpreted it to mean getting a gigantic, greasy grilled cheese sandwich, side of fries, and a beer from Melt, a local restaurant that specializes in everything that is gigantic, greasy grilled cheese goodness.

As my weight started to creep back up, there was a direct correlation between the number on the scale and my speed. I know it's said that correlation is not causation, but I knew that my additional pounds slowed me down. It may be years since I have taken any sort of science class, but I do have a basic fundamental understanding of how physics work.

December was drawing to a close, with dark winter nights transitioning into the new promise of January and the hope that comes with a new calendar, and as I reflected on the previous twelve months I knew something had to give because 2014 was just not my year.

It started out optimistically enough, but then came that second half marathon that had me walking the final four miles, and then what was supposed to be my third half marathon got cancelled. But in the end, that was okay because my training was going horribly. Cancelling the race saved me from having to officially drop out. Then there was that whole coming in last place at the Running the Bridges and walking the entire Bernie Shuffle and, well . . .

Roughly two years after I stepped on that treadmill for the very first time and decided to give running a try, I had now officially lost my running mojo. Again.

I didn't *want* to give up on running, but I was just *so* not feeling it anymore. But I was feeling fat and slow and like a big ol' phoney, fake runner.

I felt like the dreaded "J" word—a *jogger*.

All I could do was keep moving forward. One foot in front of the other for however long as it took to cross whatever proverbial finish line lay ahead on the horizon of my life. Sometimes, moving forward is the only progress that seems achievable.

That said, with any kind of goal it helps to have a focal point to maintain. Some small insignificant spot on the wall to train the eye. Something to help stay balanced, with feet feeling precarious and unsettled.

I mean trying to always maintain a positive outlook is all well and good, but sustaining that level of optimism does not come naturally to me. Sometimes my sarcastic, cynical self just needs an excuse to get her ass off the couch to go for a run. Because if I go for a run then I can feel justified in spending the rest of the day on the couch. It's all about balance, after all.

Running-related goals live in abundance: Run a certain amount of miles per year, or month, or week. Maintain a run streak of running every single day. Aim for a personal record at a particular race. I hemmed and hawed, reading over the various goals, never quite finding the one that seemed to make the most sense for me.

It was around this time, near the end of 2014, while searching for that goal, that my friend Nathan posted on Facebook about wanting to run one race per month, amounting to twelve races over the course of a year.

This wasn't the first time I had come across such a goal—my college roommate Megan had set out, and accomplished, the same goal the prior year.

Here, finally, was a goal that felt right. It wasn't based on mileage or speed. I wouldn't have to worry about how fast or slow I went. I wouldn't need to worry about fitting in a run every day or finding a way to carve 2,014 miles into the year 2014.

All I had to do was select twelve races.

Picking races as a slow runner takes far more research than I think many faster runners realize. Those speedsters can just look at the racing calendar, then look at their personal calendar, and boom. No muss, no fuss. They can be those people who show up the morning of and register without a concern about their ability to finish within the cutoff times. The fact that a cutoff time even exists is so far outside their peripheral vision, it might not even occur to them that such a thing is an issue for other runners.

Runners like me.

As a slow runner, there are a whole host of elements that need to be taken into consideration before signing up for a race. The most important of these is *how long is it going to take me to finish?*

That, more than anything, is the question that helps guide me towards finding the right race for me. Race courses don't stay open forever—they eventually have to shut them down and open the roads to normal traffic and, luckily, most racing organizations are good about posting that information on their website.

But just knowing how long the course is going to be open is only the start. I may see a race that looks and sounds perfect, thinking, *Great! The half marathon course is going to be open for four hours and it's going to take me three and a half hours to finish. I'm going to be just fine.*

Well.

The question, see, is how is that course time calculated.

This isn't a trick question, I promise. It's more sort of like if The Doctor was a race director. It's all a little wibbley-wobbley, timey-wimey when it comes to being a slow runner. Only, y'know, there's no actual mad man in a blue box waiting for you at the finish line.

When looking at course cutoffs, I'm estimating my projected finish time based on how long it will take me to get from the start line to the finish line. In other words, I'm going by chip time. The chip turns on at Point A when I cross the starting mat and turns off at Point B when I cross the finishing mat. The race organization, however, may be going by *clock time*, which starts counting down as soon as the race starts, regardless of how long it may take me to officially start the race.

In a smaller race, this isn't that big of a deal. We're talking maybe a few minutes difference between the race starting and you crossing the start line.

But in bigger races, ones that use a corral system, this works against slow runners since race etiquette states that faster and elite runners start up front with slower runners and walkers in the very back. In small races, where everyone just lines up wherever they want, it's more of an honor system thing. With big races, runners often give their projected finish time when registering and the race organizers use that number to assign corrals. Elite runners start in the first corral and the assigned positions move back from there, with slow runners and walkers being in the very last corral.

Once again, there is going to be a lag time between the official start of the race and when a runner officially starts running—only now it's going to be a much bigger lag time, possibly a significant amount of time. A significant amount of time that I now need to build into my possible finish if I'm working with a set course closure that is close to my overall finish time.

While I can certainly appreciate the desire to start out in the front or jump corrals to avoid all of that, I'm going to go ahead and tell you not to do that. There are safety reasons why slow runners line up in the back, as annoying as it may be for us sometimes. It's sort of like when you're driving on the freeway and there are a majority of cars going 70 mph and then mixed in with all the other cars are a handful going 45 mph.

Those drivers keeping their cars at a steady 70 mph are going to get frustrated at the cars going 45 mph, and they are well within their right to be frustrated. Those 45 mph cars, whether they know it or not, are disrupting the flow of traffic and the 70 mph cars are going to have to play a dangerous game of dodge 'em just to keep their pace. This could potentially cause accidents and collisions.

There is a reason why the far right lane of a highway or freeway or interstate or what have you, is often designated as the slow lane. So if you as a slow runner ever find yourself among a faster group of runners during a race (and there are many justifiable reasons why this may happen), be like those cars in the slow lane of the highway and stick to the outside of the course. This will allow the faster runners to easily move around you without disrupting the flow and speed.

I get it, too, since it happens in the back of the pack as well. Walkers are awesome. I love walkers. I have walked races myself. But walkers often walk in groups of people. Groups that stretch the entire width of the road. Some fast walkers match my speed as a slow runner and I have to zig and zag and weave my way in and out of the walkers to get myself to an open space. That said, it's also a catch-22 that we slow runners often find ourselves in on race day. We want to practice safe race etiquette by planting ourselves in the back, but we also know we are racing against the clock in a situation that works against us without really realizing it.

As I said: wibbly-wobbly, timey-wimey.

The second thing to consider is *What time does the race start?*

This might not seem like that big of a deal because all it really dictates is what time you have to wake up, right?

Wrong.

As an example: the Cleveland Marathon races are held in mid-May every year, which can be a frustrating season because the weather is still slightly unpredictable. May hovers on that line between spring and summer, which means some years it may be nice and cool and other years it's blazing hot. Like running through the corridors of Hades itself. The fact that the race ends with the runners out there on uncovered concrete for the final four miles doesn't really help with that whole exposure to the sun thing.

(See, that whole read-your-course-map-carefully thing keeps coming back!)

For those of us in the back of the pack, this means that while the race might start in the cold darkness of early morning, we're going to be out there fighting against the sun for several hours. The longer the race, the longer I am going to be exposed to the elements.

And, sure, while I'm finishing my 3:30 half marathon, there are still fast marathon runners out there working on their sub-4 hour race. So just imagine what the slow marathon runners are dealing with.

∼∼∼

So, if I was going to follow through and do this "run one race a month for the whole of 2015" thing, and I mean really do it, really commit to it, I needed to start off on the right (and left) foot.

This meant running the first of my twelve races as soon as I could.

The Commitment Day 5K is held on January 1 at various Life Time Fitness gym facilities all over the United States. I knew about it because my friend Alan had posted finish line photos from previous years of embarking on this challenge.

Oh, what's this? A race on the first day of the New Year? WELL. DON'T MIND IF I DO.

My boyfriend Ben was going out of town that weekend, meeting up with some friends down in Miami. While I was stuck suffering through Northeast Ohio snow, he was going to be hanging out in Florida.

Yes, a small part of me hated him for it.

Before dropping him off at the airport on December 31, 2014, we stopped for brunch at a little greasy spoon near his house. The kind of greasy spoon that only takes cash, a not-so-small detail that we missed before sitting down. But, that's why they have those ATMs with exuberant fees sitting near the cash register, right?

After placing our order, the waitress asked if we had any plans for New Year's Eve. Ben explained he was going to Miami for the weekend. She looked at me. "You don't mind him going alone?"

Uhhhhh. No? Should I?

When she left, Ben looked at me. "Do you want to come to Miami and hang out with my friends and go see four nights of Phish?"

I laughed. "No. I want to go to bed early tonight and go run my 5K in the morning."

He nodded. "That's what I thought."

He gets it, that whole dating a runner part of our relationship.

While I love Halloween, I'm kind of meh on New Year's Eve. I mean, I get it. Resolutions. Clean slate. It's like an annual celebration of Scarlett O'Hara's "Tomorrow is another day" mantra. Even though, technically speaking, *any* day can be a new day, there is something poetic and satisfactory in turning the calendar to January.

Except, see, the thing about New Year's Eve is that it doesn't really start until midnight, which is way past my bedtime. Cinderella turning into a pumpkin and all that.

So I usually just stay home on December 31. Sometimes that's been a result of really horrible weather and not wanting to risk a car accident just to get drunk at a party. Other times it's because I had gotten the latest *Sex and the City* season on DVD for Christmas and, y'know, PRIORITIES.

Even when I do go out, I'm the New Year's Eve guest who is asleep on my friend's couch by 10 p.m. Real crazy partier here, let me tell you.

Right, so, the Life Time Fitness gym where this race was held was about half an hour away, so I needed to add that commute into my early morning routine. The forecast didn't predict snow, but it was January and still cold outside so I layered up.

Once I got to the gym, I parked my car and headed inside. At the information desk, the clerk pointed me in the direction of the race registration. Bib numbers weren't pre-assigned, and they were simply being handed out as runners showed up. I was Lucky Number Thirteen. On the bib was a spot for me to write my name and also a line where I could write my commitment.

As I carefully wrote out *Complete one race per month in 2015*, I smiled to myself, knowing I had picked the perfect race to start my running goal.

After pinning the bib to the front of my jacket, I wandered into the gymnasium where all of the other runners were waiting and keeping warm before the gun went off. Hanging on the wall near the exit doors to the outside was a map of the course. I went over to study it, just to kind of get a feel for where I'd be running. (Not that I actually remembered any of it once I got out there but at least I was *trying* to pay more attention to course maps.)

Like the Bernie Shuffle 5K, this was a very low-key race. Other Commitment Day races at other Life Time Fitness facilities have timing chips and all of that jazz, but 2015 seemed to be the first year for this particular location and they were taking a more minimal approach. There was a clock that would be posted at the finish line, but the group running was small enough that I wasn't worried about any sort of lag time that comes with larger races.

At the designated time, the organizers opened the side doors and let us outside. After lining us up on the sidewalk, off we went.

The course took advantage of the sidewalks in and around the gym and the nearby neighborhood. After running through the parking lot down to the road, I turned along the sidewalk and found myself running parallel to the main road.

As I've said before, the past couple months I had been experimenting with walking intervals. Some of the time these were structured intervals, like when I ran the Cleveland Half Marathon the previous May. Other times, I ran until I was tired, then I walked until I wasn't tired anymore, and then I started running again.

One of the unfortunate side effects of regaining some of my weight wasn't just that the extra body mass slowed me down, but that running itself wasn't as easy. I had lost some of my endurance and was constantly struggling to regain it. Before, running three miles had been pretty easy. That is, running the whole of three miles. Now, I had to have more walking breaks. When I trained for my first half this happened but that was at longer distances.

This particular race was an event where I discovered something interesting: *people don't like being passed by a fat girl.*

I've had it happen since, but this was my first time experiencing it. I'd watch people ahead of me keep a pretty steady and consistent pace, be it walking or running, for a good long while. They were in their groove. But as soon as I passed them and was now ahead of them, suddenly their pace picked up and they'd get in the lead again. Then they'd settle back into that same consistent pace until I passed them again.

LOL. I'm sorry that my fabulously fat runner's body makes you self-conscious and all but if you want to make this some kind of game or whatever you best know who you're playing against because I will make you *work* for that lead.

In and out of the nearby neighborhood we went, around the quiet homes still sleeping in after celebrating the coming of 2015. Back up the sidewalk and through the gym's parking lot. The course took us around the back of the building to come around to the other side, where there was an inflatable arch and the finish line.

A gym employee stood right near the finish holding an iPad with a clock on it. I watched the seconds creep up. 49 minutes and 30 seconds. 49 minutes and 31 seconds.

With my eyes trained steadily on that clock, I picked up my feet and forced myself to go as fast as I could. Just finish in under 50 minutes. Just finish in under 50 minutes. Just finish in under 50 minutes.

As I crossed beneath the arch, the clock flipped over to 49 minutes and 40 seconds. I was right under 16-minute miles, 15:59 to be exact, but under 16 minutes was under 16 minutes.

I bent over at the waist to catch my breath from that final push, then gathered myself up and went into the gymnasium where they had tables with water, bananas, and chocolate milk set up. So far, my 2015 was off to a fantastic start.

When I ran my first 5K back in 2012, I had no idea what to do with my racing bibs. Throw it away? Hang it on the wall? Shove it in a drawer and forget about it until the next time I Marie Kondo the shit out of my apartment?

I didn't know if I would ever run another race after that so I didn't want to get rid of the bib, but I just was at a loss as to what to *do* with it. At the suggestion of another racing friend, I started a scrapbook. Each race gets its own page which includes the bib, any photos, and all the relevant information like race name, date, time, and all of that. Of course, all of that on its own would be boring so there are also lots of appropriately themed stickers which means I have a built-in excuse to visit my local craft store on a regular basis and spend a ridiculous amount of money. I may even buy stickers for races I'm only considering running. Like the ability to use said stickers on a scrapbook page is enough of a carrot to get me to sign up because OOOOH. SHINY. HOW CUTE ARE THOSE?!

For the Commitment Day 5K, this meant New Year's stickers but for that page I also added a slip of paper where I could keep track of all of the races I'd run that year. As I wrote the name of that morning's race on the line for January, I beamed.

One race down. Eleven more to go.

13
Walk the Talk

My friend Staci likes to call me a warrior woman.

This started several years ago when I accidentally walked six miles one afternoon. It really was an accident, as it wasn't planned, but it also wasn't a situation where I got lost. It was more like I had an errand to run and I unintentionally took the scenic route to reach my destination. And I just happened to do it on foot.

It was late summer, early fall: roughly sometime shortly before mid-September, and, with my mom's birthday coming up, my sister and I had decided that we'd treat her, and in turn my dad, to a date night by buying her a gift certificate to a local restaurant, as well as one to the independent movie theater chain here in Cleveland. My apartment in downtown Cleveland was situated roughly halfway between two of the theater locations, about a mile and a half in either direction. Given my personal preference for one location over the other, that's the theater I headed to in brand-spanking-new, comfy flip-flops that I had found on a trip to Target.

At the time I was working a job where my weekend consisted of one week day. On the one hand, this was great because it meant I could do things like go run errands at Target and not worry about all the usual crowds. On the other hand, this meant that sometimes I forgot that some small places of business operate on a slightly different schedule than their national counterparts. Like, say, a certain local independent movie theater that not only doesn't offer morning matinees, they don't even open until after noon on Fridays.

Which, of course, I didn't realize until I was knocking on a locked door at 11:30 a.m.

I could see someone in there at the register and so I get out my iPhone and look up the phone number. When they answer I explain that I'm not here for a movie, but I'd just walked a mile and a half, and I only need a gift card. Is there any way they can help?

Unfortunately not, she explains, because they don't have the computers booted up or anything like that.

Well, alrighty then.

So, I do the only thing I can do, which is turn around and head back in the direction of the mile and a half it will take me to get back to my apartment.

Halfway there I realize that while this particular location wasn't open this early, another theater, one that's a mile and a half away from my apartment but in the opposite direction, would be open. So, instead of making the turn that would take me back to my apartment, I just keep walking. I keep walking all the way to that other theater, buy the gift certificate for my mom, then walk back home.

Apartment to Theater A: one and a half miles. Theater A to Theater B: three miles. Theater B to Apartment: one and a half miles.

Six miles.

Later that evening I was in the Tremont neighborhood at a party celebrating the one-year anniversary of my friend Lauren's local business. A party that was headlined by my friend, Maura's, alt-folk and Americana band, Maura Rogers & the Bellows. It was there, standing in the streets of Cleveland on an evening that whispered of the arrival of autumn, the sounds of Americana lighting the night afire, that my friend Staci casually asked what I did that morning.

"Oh, I accidentally walked six miles."

She slowly turned her head, a look of incredulity on her face. "What?"

With a sigh, I shook my head and rolled my eyes. "I needed a gift certificate and since it was a nice day, I decided to walk to the Capitol Theatre but they were closed so then I decided to walk to Tower City Cinemas and then I walked home. It was super annoying."

Staci continued to stare at me in disbelief.

I grinned. "In flip-flops, no less."

Thus, the warrior woman nickname was born.

When it comes to walking, though, I really am kind of a warrior. This is evidenced, of course, by my refusal to run the mile in school, even though I happily walked it and would have happily walked a second mile.

Walking comes naturally to me as it does most people, I'm sure. It's how the majority of us, those who are able-bodied, navigate the world.

Walking when it comes to running did not come quite as easily.

When I first started running I used a structured program that utilized intervals. I would run for a period of time then walk for a period of time then run again. Rinse and repeat. As the program progressed, the running times would get longer as the walking times got shorter and eventually I was only running. Once I crossed that threshold any and all walking as related to running felt like cheating. It felt like a failure.

How could I call myself a runner if I *walked*?

I'd break it out, too. Break it down. Dissect the data. My first half marathon required long runs in the middle of high summer and there were times when it was just too hot to keep up a running pace. Hell, sometimes it was too hot to keep up a moderate walking pace. After, I'd come home and post on Facebook about how I completed ten miles, but I only "really" did seven or eight.

It took me a few years and several races to accept that it's okay to walk sometimes, to accept that it's really okay that I don't run entire distances or races. Whatever combination of running, walking, crawling, skipping (okay, maybe not that one) which gets me to the finish is all that matter. Ten miles is ten fucking miles regardless of the method used.

I'm not the only person who thinks that walking is legit. Race walking is an Olympic sport and has been a major Track and Field event since the late nineteenth century. Even fast runners have to walk sometimes: between Miles Twenty and Twenty-One of the Boston Marathon is Heartbreak Hill, a notorious 600-meter ascent that is challenging to even the most well-trained participants. Once I learned that Boston Marathon runners sometimes have to walk, I stopped believing that walking during a race of any distance made me any less of an athlete.

Of course, when I started, I didn't have someone like me to pass on these words of wisdom and encouragement. I didn't know anything about intervals other than that it was used as a means to an end during my Couch to 5K training. The name Jeff Galloway meant absolutely nothing to me. I didn't know that taking walking breaks during long-distance running can actually be beneficial and that runners, the fast people I think of as quote, un-quote "real" runners, often take advantage of said breaks throughout a race.

When I started running, I only walked when I absolutely needed to. Which meant I only walked when my body was basically on the verge of collapse. I have literally hobbled across finish lines because my legs and feet couldn't take it anymore. By that point, when I'm exhausted to the point of less-walking, more-shuffling, it was pretty much too late for any benefit that would come from the active recovery portion of a walking break.

Because when I get right down to it, that's really what those walking breaks are: active recovery. It's a chance for my body to recover while moving at a lower intensity, but while still keeping my heart rate up and being active. Make no mistake, walking breaks and intervals are not leisurely Sunday strolls through the park. It should still be a bit of a workout, it's just less of a workout than full-on running.

It was my Uncle Don who first introduced me to the idea of walking breaks, although I didn't know that at the time it happened. We were standing at the start line of the ConocoPhillips 10K in Houston and working on a game plan for the next 6.2 miles. He's a hard-core runner, far more athletic than I am, so I was a little surprised when he first suggested we walk up hills and through water stations. At the time, I thought he was only saying that for my benefit, knowing that this was my first 10K and that my athletic abilities were slightly behind his. Now, though, I think he was saying that because he sees the value in taking walking breaks in a race.

The 2014 Cleveland Half Marathon was the first time I really started to experiment with walking breaks, running for about 12 minutes, then walking for 3. I really was experimenting, too. That duration of interval was something I just kind of made up, and while the end for that particular race wasn't as strong as I would have liked, up until Mile Nine I was doing well with the intervals.

As I continued to run more races with walking breaks added in, and as my own endurance for running started to decline thanks to changes in my body composition (fine, whatever, I gained weight), I decided at the start of 2015 to be both more accepting of my need to sometimes walk during races and also make a concerted effort to build such walks into my runs and races. Not just walk when I felt tired, but have a specific routine that I followed.

Having also committed to running one race per month for all of 2015, I needed to start making a plan and schedule. Finding races in the warmer months was easy—I wasn't even limited to staying directly in Cleveland. Northeast Ohio has a substantial racing community, so every weekend in the spring, summer, and fall had several races I could choose from. The challenging part was locating said races that would fulfill my needs when it was less than ideal running conditions. January had been easy since there had been a race designed specifically around setting goals for the New Year, but February was going to be a bit more difficult.

My second race of the year, the SnoBall 5K, is held annually in late February in Bay Village, Ohio, a small western suburb located about fifteen miles away from downtown Cleveland. As a community, Bay Village hosts multiple races throughout the year; this would be my second one there. Like the previous race in which I had competed, the course started and ended at the Bay Village High School. The only difference this time around was that when I ran the Bay Days 5 Mile on July 4, 2013, I only had to contend with heat. Now, though, since it was February, I had to deal with the exact opposite and I spent all week watching the forecast.

The weather had been freezing cold all week so I was excited to see that it was going to be slightly warmer the weekend of the race. Of course, by "warmer" I mean temps in the 30s versus the 20s, but I'll take what I can get. What I wasn't looking forward to was the snow they were predicting. Lots and *lots* of snow.

Trust me, I know the irony of complaining about snow while living in Northeast Ohio seeing as how it, literally, comes with the territory, but whatever.

Maybe it's because I've had the fortunate well-rounded running experience of racing and training in weather of all varieties, but it would take a lot to make me even consider dropping out of a race. Granted, I don't know if all runners would call having the experience of running in snow and slush a good thing, but it's certainly made me an adaptable runner with a tough skin. Even when I briefly thought about skipping the Bernie Shuffle 5K three months before, it wasn't the weather that made me regret signing up; it was knowing I'd be running on a severe lack of sleep. Almost exactly two years before, at the 2013 St. Malachi, I had to deal with temperatures so frosty that by the time I got to the water station at the halfway mark, the waxy paper cups they used had fully formed ice crystals around the rims. Snow. Sleet. Slush. That race had it all, so when I woke up on a morning in late February 2015 and looked out my window to see a white winter wonderland of several feet, the idea of not going to the SnoBall 5K didn't even occur to me.

After layering up, I collected all of my running gear and got in the car. It was a good thing I have a tendency to leave obnoxiously early, because the roads hadn't yet been cleared, which meant it was a slow and slippery going as I navigated my car across the fifteen very slick miles to the Bay Village High School.

Despite the weather, the SnoBall 5K had several hundred participants that year, many of whom were already at the high school when I arrived. Packet pick-up was inside the hallway outside of the gymnasium and pockets of people were camped out on the bleachers, trying to stay dry and warm for as long as possible before needing to head outside to the start line. I found the registration tables and checked in. After taking my race shirt back to my car, I headed back into the school to join everyone else as we waited for the call to line up.

As any who've tried it know, running in snow is not for the faint of heart. I don't even mean just dealing with frigid temperatures and trying to balance dressing warmly enough to not freeze to death while also making sure the body doesn't overheat. That's all taken care of before even stepping outside. No, just the physical act of running in snow and especially *on* snow, is a mental and physical challenge. Your muscles get used in a completely different way than they did when running in non-winter and, for me at least, it's hard to get into that running zone where I can tune everything else out because I have to constantly be aware of the ground in front of me lest I slip on ice and fall, thus putting myself out of running commission for weeks or even months.

Around the second mile, it was all starting to catch up with me. I was utterly exhausted from what felt like hours and hours of walking in snow and, because of said snow, I was absolutely freezing. It was falling hard and fast, making it difficult to see, and the thought that I still had a mile to go exhausted me even more.

I was also in last place and not even trying to pretend otherwise. In other races when I've been one of the stragglers at the end, I usually try to at least put in a good effort: I stick to my intervals and run when I can. I want to finish a race knowing that even if I didn't necessarily do my very best or do as well as I would have liked, I at least gave it my all.

With the SnoBall 5K, woo boy that was so not happening. My desire to not be out in the snow and cold was so extreme that there were multiple moments where I wanted to turn around, go to the police car following me, and ask if he would mind driving me back to the Bay Village high school because I had officially hit my limit.

But I didn't. Even though I wanted to. *Really* wanted to. This was pretty much on par with what I was feeling during those final four miles at the 2014 Cleveland Half, only this time I was cold and freezing and shivering.

In this instance, the one unexpected benefit to being in the back is that I never had to guess where I was going on the course. Because the streets hadn't been plowed, the runners in front of me had all beaten down a slushy path in the snow.

Another unexpected benefit was that it gave me time to mentally work on the Ignite! Fitness presentation that I would be giving at the upcoming FitBloggin 2015 conference in Denver. FitBloggin is an annual conference that focuses on health and fitness with a vast online community of participants. I discovered FitBloggin through some social media networks and was so disappointed when I realized the 2013 conference was going to be the same weekend as my sister's wedding. (She has forgiven me for a lot of things, but skipping out on her nuptials would not have gone over well.) 2014 was the first year I attended. At the Keynote Address on the Friday night of the conference, FitBloggers get up on a stage to give Ignite! Presentations. These last five minutes each with accompanying auto-forwarding slides. The presentations cover a wide range of topics and are voted on by the FitBloggin community.

In anticipation of the 2015 conference, I submitted an Ignite! presentation that covered the topic of being in the back of the pack. It was titled *It's Not Last Place, it's Running with a Police Escort*, inspired by the photo I took of myself at the Running the Bridges, with a cop car over my shoulder.

A few weeks before the SnoBall 5K I found out that my topic was one of the ones selected. The conference wasn't until that June, but I knew that was going to come quickly and I hadn't yet given that much thought to my presentation.

Considering I was currently slowly trudging through the snow, in last place, this seemed like as good a time as any to start giving this some thought.

Near the end, the main road splintered and the path followed a slight curve back behind the school, continuing to the finish line.

Up ahead I saw the familiar black finish clock in the middle of the high school stadium. The finish line itself was along the track which hadn't been cleared. Because of course it hadn't. Why would they clear the high school track in the middle of *February* for fuck's sake?

As I turned the corner and headed towards the finish, I heard a car horn behind me. I turned around and the police officer who had been following for the past three miles gave me a thumbs-up sign before driving past.

Police escort, yo. That's what I'm talking about.

I slogged through the snow towards the finish, attempting to match the established footprints of the runners who had finished before me. Then, after finishing, I slogged through the snow back to the high school. A set of tables was set up in the middle of the gymnasium piled high with gleaming bright aluminum food warmers. My stomach growled with hungry anticipation.

In my desire to be finished, I had completely forgotten that the SnoBall 5K included a post-race pancake breakfast and awards ceremony.

My experience with post-race award ceremonies is pretty limited. I think in all my time I've seen only a handful out of over twenty races. Most races don't wait for everyone to finish before handing out awards, which, I mean, I totally understand. The winners of the awards are always the fast runners, the ones who finished in record time. Literally, in some instances, where they manage to be so fast they set a new course record. These are the runners who finished early and I can totally understand why it makes more sense to hand those awards out while other runners are still running rather than make the winners just hang out for a significant amount of time until everyone gets back. Depending on the race and the runners on the course, they could be waiting at least an hour.

So I certainly always appreciate when a racing organization makes the effort to make sure *all* runners have finished before starting the awards ceremony. And, it turns out, if you're going to convince the faster runners to stick around until those of us in the back of the pack return, it helps to have more than just the usual banana and chocolate milk waiting at the finish line.

Like, say, hot, delicious pancakes slathered in maple syrup and butter. Yup, that'll definitely do the trick.

14
Trust the Process

A couple of weeks after the SnoBall 5K, it was once again time for the annual St. Malachi race. While Northeast Ohio obviously has races in January and February (I just ran one per month), St. Malachi is often considered the unofficial start to the racing season in Cleveland.

At the beginning of the year, when I committed to running one a month, there were certain races I knew I'd be remiss if I *didn't* run them as part of this goal. St. Malachi was one of those races. 2015 also marked the thirty-fifth anniversary of the race and in honor of this milestone, there was going to be a special finisher's medal. Not that I needed additional encouragement or anything, my "Will Run For Bling" stance clearly ingrained, but still.

St. Malachi also fit in perfectly with my training plan. As of Monday, February 23, 2015, I was officially back in training mode, this time for what would be my third half marathon. Not only would I be running my third half marathon, but I'd be running it as an Ambassador. As an official Ambassador, in exchange for my own free race entry, I got to blog about my training experience, give someone else a chance to run for free, and promote the race across all the usual social media platforms.

I should have been excited about this. I was going to be running my *third* half marathon and represent both the back of the pack and the city that I love.

Me. Third half. Numero Tres. Three times a charm, right?

Only, I was actually dreading it. Dreading the early morning alarm clock calls. Dreading the sacrifice to my social calendar as I planned early Friday night outings to fit in even earlier Saturday morning runs. I had already gone through this all before. *Twice.* I knew the long road ahead, I knew the hard work that would be required and the blood and sweat and tears that would come (hopefully not literally, but after my second half marathon, anything was possible).

My last half marathon, the 2014 Cleveland Half, left me feeling dejected, and then the whole cancellation of the second Cleveland Rock 'N' Roll Half. Add in that a May half marathon means starting training in February. In Cleveland, this is not a month that is typically kind to runners. Limited sunlight means running indoors on the dreadmill or running in the dark, neither of which is my favorite way of getting in my training runs.

Being a slow runner only complicated matters. My first training run on the program was for three miles. For a seasoned long-distance runner, three miles is a pretty minor distance to tackle for an early morning run. But because of my speed, I have to build in extra time into my mornings to make sure I give myself enough of a buffer to get the run in and still get to work on time. Someone who averages a 10-minute mile only needs half an hour of their morning. For me, I needed 45 minutes on a good day. But because I hadn't been running as much and had lost some of my base, I was starting from scratch in some ways, which meant I would be slower than usual and/or would be adding in more walking breaks, so my three mile run was going to take something closer to an hour to complete. That wasn't even counting the time it would take me to get dressed in weather-appropriate gear and, oh yeah, actually wake up enough to function to the point of even being able to go run three miles.

Take that, then multiply it by multiple runs over multiple weeks and, oh yeah, add in extra miles each week, building up the long runs, and add in additional early mornings for cross-training.

So, yeah. Not looking forward to this whole "training" thing.

Training for a half marathon is similar to any journey. There will be obstacles and detours. There will be hills and valleys (sometimes even literal ones) that need to be climbed. Things won't always go as planned no matter how expensive a GPS you own. Training is sort of like dealing with a GPS that hasn't been updated in a while, unaware of road closures or lane changes. Following such a GPS can lead to frustration, as you're forced to quickly maneuver and figure out a different route to your destination.

Focusing on the process means the destination is more likely to be a blip than a boom. And the end result becomes just that: the final data point in a long line of other data points. Which, really, makes the most sense out of everything else. With a half marathon training program, that's something like twelve to sixteen weeks during which hundreds of miles are covered. Literally, *hundreds* of miles all told.

That totally blows my mind, even now. To think that over the course of a couple of months, I can run that many miles and yet so much focus and effort is put on those final 13.1 miles (or 26.2 for those that run full marathons).

Obviously the goal race, the one for which you put in all that training, is important. It's the reason I am training to begin with, but putting all my attention on that end result, those final 13.1 miles, that bright blue finish line, makes me anxious. I put so much pressure on the outcome of that race, on those particular 13.1 miles, that I somehow lose sight of those hundreds of miles that come first in the weeks and months leading up to the race. Why do I find those other miles, of which there are so many more, somehow less important, less significant? Those miles are the ones that prepare my mind and prepare my body to rock those final 13.1 miles come race day. I wouldn't have successfully crossed all of those finish lines without those training miles under my belt.

Five of those miles were going to be completed at the St. Malachi.

It's probably just a coincidence, but the St. Malachi always seems to line up perfectly with my training plan. Even when I've picked a shorter spring race, the two mile option at St. Malachi is like a square peg in a square hole on my calendar.

The first two weeks of my training had gone well, although, I had to add in an extra rest day because I'd been battling a cold. Admittedly, I probably wouldn't have let myself be sidelined because of a few sniffles, but I just felt so run down, and since I was already not digging being in training mode, I took what excuses presented themselves.

It's impossible to predict what the weather will be like when St. Malachi rolls around. In 2013, I battled hail and snow. A couple years before I started running, it was a bright sunny day, warm enough that wearing short sleeves wasn't crazy.

That year, it was a mostly typical late winter, early spring day. It had rained the night before but when I woke up on race morning the sky was dry, although it was a little chilly and I was going to need to wear a jacket. Underneath, I had a green Guinness shirt and was also sporting green sparkly shamrocks in my hair and coordinating knee-high socks.

I don't really get St. Patrick's Day as a holiday—all-day drinking doesn't appeal to me and never has, not even in college—but I have fake red hair and look good in green, so it's one of the easier races to get in the spirit and dress up for. Like Miranda said in an episode of *Sex and the City*, "Anybody can be Irish with the right colorist."

The race starts on the corner of Detroit and West 25th, two major streets in the neighborhood. This corner also marks the home of the actual St. Malachi Church, which the race represents. Before the race, their basement Fellowship area is open for the runners to hang out in while they wait.

A couple of the Cleveland Marathon Ambassadors were also running in this race, and as I stood inside, I kept updating my Facebook feed to see if anyone was posting their own location. Because the weather wasn't too bad, lots of runners were also waiting outside all around the church property so trying to find someone was a bit tricky. Megan also tends to run St. Malachi on an annual basis, but I've only managed to connect with her one year and even then it was purely by accident. But at least I knew her, so when I saw her standing in the same pocket as me I was able to recognize her. I hadn't as of yet met any of the other Ambassadors in person, I only had social media profiles to go by.

Mary, then social media director for the Cleveland Marathon, mentioned she was on the back end of the church so I went outside and headed up to try to find her. Somehow, against all likelihood, I found

Mary and we stood around chatting and she introduced me to her friends.

As we started to line up near the west entrance of the Veteran's Memorial Bridge—also known as the Detroit-Superior Bridge—I mentioned to Mary that I had started doing intervals. She said she was a big fan of those and did one minute of running followed by one minute of walking.

"Do you want to run with me?" she asked.

"Oh," I said, "I'm slow."

"That's okay! I am, too."

We stood next to each other in the crowd, near the back. When the gun went off, the crowd surged forward, carrying us with it.

The Veteran's Memorial Bridge is about half a mile long and four lanes wide. Because it's close to the church, it's a natural starting point for this race and I always love watching the crowd take over the whole bridge right from the start. It's just a moving sea of green folks spread the entire width and breadth of the bridge.

Thing was, Mary's idea of "slow" was much faster than mine, and while I tried to keep up with her intervals as long as I could, we had barely made it over the bridge before I told her I had to slow down. Between the quicker pace and the cold I was battling, I was having a hard time catching my breath.

It's like in television shows and movies when the unathletic protagonist decides to start running and turns to those super fit neighbors next door, assuming it'll be totes easy to join them on a morning run. Two minutes in, our protagonist is standing on the side of the road, bent over at the waist, panting, waving the neighbors ahead: "Just . . . go . . . on . . . without . . . me."

Yeah. It was just like that.

As Mary ran ahead, I slowed to a walk as the rest of the back of the pack moved around me.

Because I had started way faster than I should have, I spent the rest of the race struggling to find my groove. That first half mile at a pace far speedier than my body was ready to run made for a very long remaining four and a half miles.

After crossing the bridge, the course turns left and starts to head towards Lake Erie. The course ran parallel to the Shoreway, although this time on the actual ground beneath, past First Energy Stadium, the Great Lakes Science Center, and the Rock 'N' Roll Hall of Fame and Museum.

The halfway point of the race was the Burke Lakefront Airport, a very small airport situated right, as its name suggests, on the lake. Along with being the halfway point, it was also our first and only water stop. The course took us through their horseshoe driveway then we headed back where we came, this time going behind the home of the Cleveland Browns.

By now I was walking more than I had planned, but my legs still burned from their earlier attempt at a speed outside my ability. But I tried to run as much as I could as I continued to follow the course, sticking to my intervals as best as I could.

At this point, the finish was still another half mile or so away, and at the next turn, I was directed to go down a long hill. Runners who had already finished were walking up the hill as I bolted towards the finish.

Running downhill? Magical. Fucking magical I tell you. It doesn't matter how slow my run up until then has been. Hell, I could be out there having the worst possible run ever, but as soon as I hit a downhill section I turn into a fucking Olympian. (In my mind, at least.) The wind at my back, I am picking up so much speed and making up for lost time, might as well just hand me that gold medal right now.

Of course, I'm not exactly the most coordinated individual out there and so I have to be careful and not give fully into my capabilities because I would be that clumsy idiot who trips over her feet and doesn't run down the hill so much as *roll* down it and that's not quite the photo finish I'm aiming for here.

At the bottom of the hill, the course turns left to a tenth of a mile stretch of flat road.

When I made that final turn and set my sights on the finish line up ahead, I also noticed the two women standing on the other side of the blue mat. They each held the last few remaining finisher's medals. I'm talking maybe five total medals between the two of them.

So, here's the thing with finisher's medals. Unless it's a race that sets a registration cap, there's really no guarantee a runner will get their medal. This is a sad reality that unfairly affects many in the back of the pack. While I've always been fortunate enough to receive my medal, I've heard stories from friends who haven't been so lucky.

As long as a race allows for same-day registrations, there's always a chance they will run out. A racing organization has to order medals in advance and while they can use whatever tools they have available to guesstimate how many medals to order, there's still a chance they'll underestimate.

Finisher's medals are first come first serve.

Which is all well and good, except when a bunch of front and middle of the pack runners show up the day of the race and decide to run. They finish first. They get their medals. The more medals they receive, the less that are available to those runners in the back who are still working their way through the course.

That race, I got lucky. As the volunteer handed me my medal, I made a quick count and I knew there were still runners behind me who might not be quite as lucky. It was going to be close for sure. As someone who knows she'll never win a racing medal for coming in first (or second, or third), the finisher's medals mean a lot to me, just as they no doubt mean a lot to all of the other runners in the back of the pack. I can't even imagine how devastating it would be to put in the training, to show up on race day, to complete the race, and then not get a medal just because I was too slow and didn't get to the finish line fast enough. I mean, hello. Look at everything I did a few months ago just to get that Bernie medal. Finisher's medals are legit serious business. Don't be getting between me and my bling.

I finished, but I didn't finish fast, averaging close to 17-minute miles. I started out way too fast in the beginning and my body just couldn't keep up. Even if I wasn't, y'know slow, I don't know if I'd have been able to keep up with that pace. Then there was that whole hacking up a lung thing and I was pretty much doomed from the start.

Over the next couple of days my cold progressed and my body was starting to feel tired. And not just normal tired. Not the tired that comes with training and early morning runs and late night workouts. This was exhausted. Lethargic. Fatigued. Finally, I sucked it up and went to the doctor who advised me to consider taking a week off from my training.

I was early enough in my training that missing a week's worth of workouts wouldn't set me back too far. But, still. A whole week? I mean, what if I take off and my body just, like, *forgets* how to run?

The other option was to fight through it. To keep going, to push myself through the workouts and the runs, no matter how horrible I felt, no matter how tired and sick my body was.

I decided to listen to my body, and the doctor, and take the week off. If I was later in my training, I don't know if I would have made the same decision but this particular time it was the right choice.

So now, with three races now done, I was a quarter of the way through my 2015 racing goal. Only one more race stood between me and the half marathon.

15
The Hero's Journey

For the past couple miles I have had one mantra repeating itself, anxiously increasing in both speed and volume with each loop:

I'm pretty sure I'm lost.

During races, my mind goes a million miles a minute. Some thoughts are good, like when I'm jamming to my running playlist and my power song comes on and I'm just all YEAH LET'S DO THIS THING. (I want to be all hip and cool and tell you that my power song is something old school like Survivor's "Eye of the Tiger," but it's the Nicki Minaj version of "Anaconda." #Sorrynotsorry.)

Moments like that are good. But the flip side of that is when I'm a mile into a five-mile run and my brain all of a sudden wakes up and is like WHAT THE FUCK ARE YOU DOING?! Why are we running? Why are we out in the [insert: rain, snow, cold, other miscellaneous forms of precipitation] running when we could be inside, warm under the covers? My feet are yelling at me, my body is yelling at me, my brain is yelling at me and I just kind of want to give in and go home but I still have four miles to go and OMG I hate my life.

Those moment are less good. But if there's one thought I do not, under any circumstance, want to have pass across the fog of my

167

consciousness mid-race, it's the vague notion that I may very well have drifted off course.

But nevertheless here I was: hot, exhausted, and seven miles into a ten-mile race with absolutely no idea where I was going.

When I first committed to running one race a month for all of 2015, there were certain races that I knew I was going to run no matter what, like last month's St. Malachi 5 Mile. Other months I was playing by ear, not sure what I'd be running until it got closer and I had a better idea of what my training would be like.

Just as St. Malachi easily fit into the beginning portion of my half marathon training, the April Hermes 10 Miler fit in perfectly near the end of my training.

Named for the Greek god who acts as a messenger between mortals and those on Mount Olympus, the Hermes 10 Miler began in 2005 as a race designed to help those runners training for half and full marathons, including the Cleveland Marathon.

As the name suggests, long runs are, uh, long. When training for a 5K, a long run might not all be that long, but as race distances increase, these runs live up to their name. Like most half marathon training plans, mine tops off at ten miles, which conveniently coincided with the Hermes 10 Miler. Additionally, with the half marathon in May and Hermes in April, I was able to my meet my April race commitment, get in a long run, and get some bling.

When I started my half marathon training in late February, I wasn't feeling confident or ready to take on the challenges ahead. But as I logged my miles and watched my progress I realized I had an opportunity to PR. So far, all signs pointed to the fact that I'd be able to run a faster half marathon than I did the very first time I tackled the distance back in 2013.

This information was gathered from all my long runs, and the Hermes 10 Miler would be the real test. At ten miles, it was close enough to a half marathon distance that I knew whatever pace and time I pulled out on that day would be a good indicator of how race day would go a couple weeks later.

That morning, I woke up early and headed over to the race site, the familiar Edgewater Park. The race was starting on the upper level, and I managed to get lucky and find a spot in the small lot. Packet pick-up had been at a local running store a few days before, so all I needed to do was show up.

I had a few friends running this race but, as always, with so many people, it's difficult to stay organized and find people. The breeze right off the lake made for a chilly morning and I was glad I wore my jacket. The bib was pinned right on the outside.

I found myself in last place as soon as the gun went off and we all started running. It was going to be a long morning and I had ten miles to cover, so there was no reason to worry about my place or pace right at the very beginning. I started doing my intervals, alternating set periods of running and walking, the little voice embedded in my running app telling me when it was time to run or walk.

The course started at the upper level of Edgewater Park near the pavilion, then looped around the walking path, and then went down towards the main road, which fed into a residential neighborhood.

Waiting at the entrance to the neighborhood was the police escort that would be following me for the majority of the race.

The middle of the pack tends to keep a consistent pace, everyone matching each other stride for stride. In the back it's more haphazard, everyone running their own race, their own pace. Because of my run-walk intervals, there are times when I'll surge ahead of someone only to fall behind them when I switch to walking. There was one such woman at the Hermes 10 Miler. For the first few miles, we were constantly trading off on who was in last place. It wasn't some unspoken thing between the two of us, simply a matter of our own running and walking styles. Eventually, though, with my intervals I managed to pull far enough ahead to secure a spot that was second to last.

Spring weather in Cleveland can be unpredictable and the jacket I had been wearing at the start of the race now left me feeling over-heated. It took an awkward few minutes and several run-walk-run rotations to unpin my bib from the front of my jacket so I could re-pin it to the front of my shirt.

The course took us in, out, and around the ritzy neighborhood right on Lake Erie, with gorgeous views of the water and palatial private homes with fences all around the property. Admittedly, I may have used my walking intervals to window-shop the large homes I will never,

ever be able to afford, but THEY ARE JUST OH SO PRETTY TO LOOK AT.

At Mile Six, the back of the pack was made up of me, that other woman, and the police escort closely following her. By now there were other police cars out on the road to open up the streets again and we were now told to move to the sidewalk.

Sigh.

Okay.

I may be horrible about reading course maps in advance, but I always read course time limits and I knew that this race specifically said that as long as a runner was below an 18-minute average they could stay on the road. At 16-minute miles, I was well below that, yet they still decided to move us onto the sidewalk, which is y'know, kind of not cool. Oh sure, just let me dodge these suburban residents doing their Saturday morning boutique shopping. I know I'm slow but goddamnit, that day I was not *that* slow.

This is another one of those challenges that slow runners face that fast runners don't and I'm always mindful of finish times and course limits; it's exasperating to go out of my way to sign up for races and keep those time limits, only to have it change on race day. But, whatever.

Things started to get a little complicated around Mile Seven, when the course started to turn back towards Edgewater Park. I know this park pretty well. I've covered many, many, *many* miles there, and have run multiple races that have used the park's paths as the course. This meant I knew there was no way in hell there was enough ground to get another three miles out of this park.

Enough time had passed since the start of the race that most people were already finished, so the entire park—including the path those of us in the back were still using—was full of runners milling around. People, bright shiny medals hanging around their necks, walked haphazardly, in all directions as they worked their way through the crowd to their parked cars.

Trying to maintain the course at this point was getting increasingly difficult, but I just stayed on the park's path as best I could and kept an eye out for volunteers and course markers. After going on another loop of the upper level of the park, we were dumped back out onto the street.

This particular area of the city has been going through a lot of changes in recent years and I was less familiar with the new landscape. There literally were no other runners around for about a mile in either direction of me.

It was around this point in the race that I legitimately began to worry I was lost. The course wasn't well marked. Or, well, maybe it was well marked, but it wasn't well thought out. So I'd be running along a stretch of sidewalk, eyes constantly shifting around trying to find an orange course marker, and my little brain would be saying *This can't be right, this can't be right* over and over again until, finally, that orange course marker appeared. And then I'd be running along that stretch of sidewalk, once again looking for the next marker, once again repeating *This can't be right, this can't be right.*

The course itself was just confusing as hell, and because it's just me out there and because it's a Saturday morning and all the non-runners were home sleeping or out brunching (lucky bastards) all I could do was keep running and hope I was running in the right direction.

As I started to run up Detroit Avenue, I knew I had to be closing in on the finish line, or at least closing in on the park. At Mile Nine I breathed a sigh of relief when I saw a policeman standing at the entrance to a newly developed neighborhood. In fact, I was so happy to see him I waved and he waved back. Across the street I heard a commotion loud enough to infiltrate my earbuds and when I looked over, I saw an old woman in a wheelchair shouting and cheering me on.

Have I mentioned that I fucking love this city?

As I turned the corner into the neighborhood, the policeman raised his index finger. One mile left. With a grin, I raised mine and kept running.

Here the committee had been a little more generous with the markers, which was good, because the course now consisted of a lot of twists and turns around new apartment buildings and town homes. But eventually the course ran towards the tunnel that would take me underground and back to Edgewater Park.

Exiting the tunnel, I realized I had completely overestimated just how close the tunnel was from the rest of the park. Seeing the finish line flag on the furthest side of the park, I estimated I still had about half a mile left. All I could do was keep running.

The tunnel opened to a long concrete ramp that zigged and zagged down, eventually connecting with Edgewater Park's walking path. As I followed the curve of the course towards the finish line, I spotted my parents waiting on a picnic bench near the perimeter.

I untied my jacket sleeves from around my waist and tossed it in the general direction of my parents. It landed softly on the grass a few feet in front of them. "Bring it to the finish!" I shouted as I picked up my pace.

(Later, at brunch, my mom told me that when my dad picked it up he said that the jacket was soaking wet with sweat.)

Several yards ahead of me, the big black flag that marked the end waved in the breeze, the words FINISH written in white. Those runners fast enough to finish before me were able to run under an inflatable arch, an arch that was already being taken down by the time that I finished.

Right there, right at the end, I felt this surge in my legs and *sprinted* for that finish line. All those walking intervals built into my race assisted in preserving my energy and endurance

Out of the corner of my eye I saw one of the race workers clapping and cheering my last push of the race and after I crossed the finish line, he came over and gave me a high five. While someone put a finisher's medal around my neck, he personally brought over a small carton of chocolate milk and banana from the pile of post-race refreshments.

Ten miles, 2 hours, and 41 minutes later, I finished the Hermes 10 Miler with an average mile time of 16:07. For a race of this distance, that was absolutely unheard of for me. This meant that I legitimately had an opportunity to get a Personal Record at my upcoming half marathon.

16

Three Times
a Charm?

It was finally here.

May 17, 2015.

Race day. For my *third* half marathon.

Several months before I had found out I had been selected as a 2015 Cleveland Marathon Ambassador; to say that I was surprised by this is an understatement. After all, I am slow. So slow that I've come in last place at more than one race. I'm also fat. Who the hell wants a slow, fat loser representing them at a major racing event?

The thing about this city is that we love a lovable loser. I mean, hello. Just look at our sports teams. (Well, okay, I mean, except for that whole 2016 NBA Championship thing which was, like, THE. BEST. DAY. EVER. But ignore that and let's, instead, look at the previous fifty-two years of Cleveland sports.) It turns out I was the perfect person to pick to be an Ambassador.

The Friday before the race was a busy one, with both packet pick-up and a swanky V.I.P. party. After spending the past weeks and months following their training programs—and having them following mine—this was going to be the first time I actually met any of my fellow Ambassadors in person and, to be perfectly honest, I was *super* nervous. They are all fast and some are triathletes and Iron(wo)men. But they were warm, friendly, and completely accepting of my speed. Like my readers, they had been following my training on my blog and knew that I was aiming for a PR at Sunday's race. Before leaving for the night we all made a plan to meet before the start of the race.

Sunday morning I was up early and quickly got ready. I'd followed my usual routine of putting my clothes out the night before, so everything was there waiting. This included a bright pink headband that said *What I lack in speed I make up for in cute.*

ALRIGHT, BITCHES. LET'S DO THIS THING.

Parking can always be a little tricky for big races because many of the roads downtown Cleveland are closed early for the race, so it can be a bit of a scramble just to get into the city, let alone find somewhere to keep your car. My boyfriend, who was not running that day, offered to wake up equally as early and drive me to the start line (or as close as he could get).

He is so totally a keeper.

Since I would be running slow and it was going to take me a few hours to complete the 13.1 miles ahead of me, he would still have plenty of time to get back to my apartment and go back to sleep before coming to get me at the finish line.

After he dropped me off, I headed in the direction of the Ambassadors agreed-upon meet-up spot. Soon I was joined by the others, and after a round of photos, hugs, and wishes of good luck, we all separated and went to line up in our assigned corrals.

Cleveland races often utilize a live tracking system that allows friends and family to get real-time updates of a runner's progress at certain points along the course. In the past, I had signed up my parents and my sister so they'd be able to know how I was doing without needing to come all the way into the city to watch. For the 2015 race, I also signed myself up for my own tracking.

I knew I was assigned to one of the last corrals, the one right before the walkers. Because I was so far away from the start line, there was going to be that expected lag time, which meant I, once again, couldn't really gauge my time and pace using the clocks along the route. The tracking system would send me a text, which was the best way to know how I was doing mid-race. That's a pro-tip from me to all the slow runners out there. You're welcome.

In typical spring fashion, there was a light smattering of sprinkles that added an unexpected chill to the early morning air. Then in one unexpected rush, the gunmetal grey sky above opened and the rain started. Many runners scurried off the course, hoping to gain tempo-rary shelter under the awnings of the buildings along the way. I stayed where I was, standing in the middle of Ontario Street, eyes raised as I watched the overcast clouds. Then, again, in typical spring weather fashion, the rain ceased just as quickly as it started, leaving us all a little bit wetter and a little bit chillier.

Someone said hello and I looked to my left and saw Debi, one of the Cleveland Ambassadors, standing beside me. A Northeast Ohio native, Debi now lives in Florida and comes up in the spring for the big race. We started chatting, looking out over the sea of runners ahead of us.

Debi was nervous about running today. *Really* nervous. When she took up running again after an injury, she made a promise to herself that she would not run in rain. Running when it's wet and slick out only increased her risk of slipping and falling and putting herself out of commission once again and she just couldn't take that chance. Her mitigation against another running injury is so strong that there have been times down in Florida when she has been registered for a local 5K and the morning of the race she would go pick up her shirt and bib, then turn around and go right back home because of the rain.

As we stood in our corral way in the back, Debi confided that this short downpour was making her consider skipping the race. Even though she was here, all ready to go, her fears about falling were height-ened thanks to Mother Nature. She went on to explain that her training hadn't been as focused as she would have liked and so that, coupled with the rain, had her on the proverbial fence.

I listened to her, grateful to lend an ear to a fellow slow runner at the start time. After thinking about it for a few seconds, I pointed out that Debi didn't have to *run* the half marathon if it made her that nervous. Walking was, and always is, a perfectly acceptable alternative, would cover the same ground, and would get her to the very same finish line when all was said and done. I mean she was already here, thousands of a miles from home, dressed, bib on, and ready to go. It honestly seemed like at this point, it would take far more energy to turn around and go home. She'd have to walk all the way to her car, which was probably parked near the finish line half a mile away, and then it would take forever for her to even get out of the city, so she might as well stick around and just do this thing. Hell, at the very least, she'd get a great workout in. Debi smiled and thanked me, agreeing that if nothing else she could always just walk. She moved away from me to find her spot in the corral and we anxiously waited for our turn to start.

They say the first mile is a liar. Well, okay, they say that, but so do I. The first mile is a liar. The first mile is probably one of the toughest miles out of any run no matter the distance. Whatever happens, a runner cannot allow that first mile to dictate the rest of their run. It makes running seem difficult, even impossible. My legs are tired and not warmed up enough. My feet feel like blocks of concrete. The first mile makes me feel like I hate running and on this particular day, as soon as I crossed the threshold and was officially headed for that blue mat 13.1 miles away, that first mile made me question my sanity.

Seriously. What the fuck had I been thinking signing up for another half marathon? Am I some kind of masochist? Was last year's half not enough proof that this is just sheer torture? What kind of crazy person gives up a Sunday morning to go running for thirteen miles?!

But then, it's like Oh. Well hello there Mile Two. I'm actually starting to feel like I've found my groove now so, y'know, just forget all that stuff I said a mile ago. I LOVE RUNNING. RUNNING IS AWESOME.

Mile Three turned the corner onto Abbey Avenue and I was yet again running down the streets where all of my friends live, although those lucky non-running bastards were still asleep. Being people who don't voluntarily pay money to run races, they've told me they only ever know it's marathon weekend when signs start going up on their street indicating they have to move their cars. For a neighborhood where everyone has street parking, this is a big pain in the ass, as they pretty much lose their normal spots right in front of their apartments.

Sorry guys. You know you still love me.

Four miles in, I decided that run-walk-run intervals were just, like, the most amazingest, bestest thing in the entire world. I was running for 30 seconds, walking for 45 seconds, and while that didn't seem like a long time, those short bursts of running were enough to let me really pick up my pace. My endurance was even—I wasn't running until I was too tired and then slowly walking until I felt rested. Those rest breaks were already built in and the method kept me feeling energized the whole time.

As I passed the marker for Mile Five, it occurred to me that if I had signed up for the 10K, I'd already be almost done.

Yeah. That's not really a good thought to have less than halfway into a half marathon. Actually, I'm pretty sure that's the worst thing to be thinking less than halfway into a half marathon.

As soon as I passed the 10K mark, I pulled my phone out of my armband. The text that came through said that I was right on target to finish in 3:30 and my current pace was around 16-minute miles. For sake of comparison, my first half, back in 2013, I had averaged 16:37 per mile with a final time 3:37:53.

This meant that I was right on target for that PR.

From here on out I had to rely on my phone's clock to know how I was doing, but since the text gave an estimated time of arrival based on the other data points, as long as I was at the finish line by 10:39 a.m., I'd be golden.

Typical of wonky Cleveland weather, the morning started off a little chilly, with the rain helping cool things off, and now the sun was starting to shine brightly and the moisture in the air was creating that horrible weather phenomenon known as humidity.

Luckily, the spectators along the course recognized what it must be like to run in such conditions and around Mile Seven there was a woman who had set up her sprinkler in the middle of the road for all of us runners to run through.

I really, really, really love this city.

Mile Eight ran through the Gordon Square neighborhood, a quaint district with lots of boutique shops and a gorgeous renovated art deco–style movie theater. The level of spectators can be somewhat hit or miss along the course: since we are often running on major roads and freeways it's not super easy for watchers to find a viewing spot. But when we run through residential neighborhoods like this one, the sidewalks are packed. One of the spectators recognized me from a storytelling event I had done over a year before and for about half a second I felt like the most famous person ever.

Halfway through Mile Eight I had to make the dreaded stop at a porta potty. And then came Mile Nine. Oh Mile Nine, you old foe you.

Last year, Mile Nine was about the location when my ankle officially quit and I was forced to walk the remaining four miles of the course. Mile Nine is also the start of what I still consider the longest four miles ever, whether I am hobbling along or running at a nice clip. Mile Nine is the entrance to half marathon hell itself.

I pulled my phone out of my armband for a time check. That PR was still achievable but it was going to be very, very close. But, it's okay. Even if I finished in 3:37:52, it will still count as a PR.

All I could do was keep going. As much as possible I tried to ignore the blazing hot sun and the amount of sweat dripping off of me. It was Mile Ten. That means I only had a 5K left. That was it, just a 5K. I've run, like, a *million* of those. And I tried really, really hard to ignore the humidity.

Humidity that had managed to drastically slow me down as indicated by my time check at Mile Eleven when it was clear that I was *not* going to PR today.

Around Mile Twelve the heat and humidity really started to get to me and I decided that I was never, ever, ever, running a half marathon again. Half marathons are stupid. I mean, really. 13.1 miles? What the fuck is up with that point one? Who thought up that one? And why are 5Ks and 10Ks named after their metric units, and halfs and fulls go by miles? That does it, it's not just half marathons. All running is dumb and stupid and the people who run are equally dumb and stupid and I don't want other people to think I'm also dumb and stupid, so no more half marathons for me. Nope. No siree.

Oh, oh! That's the marker for Mile Thirteen waving like a gorgeous blue flag against the gorgeous blue sky. Only point one to go!

JUST KEEP RUNNING. JUST KEEP RUNNING. JUST KEEP RUNNING.

I ran down the Shoreway ramp onto Lakeside, speeding up my intervals as much as I could. Even with the finish line in sight, I wanted to stick to my routine. It had gotten me this far, feeling strong and confident, and I'd see it through to the end.

As I crossed the finish line on my third half marathon I felt completely overwhelmed. Not just at even finishing my third half, but finishing it feeling so alive. Last year I practically had to crawl across but this time, thanks to the Galloway Method, I had the endurance to push myself even right there at the end. Boom, bitch.

Gathering some post-race grub, I checked my phone for my final text alert. 3:46:31. Nine minutes stood between me and that PR. I had aimed for 3:30, but anything faster than my first half marathon would have counted.

The thing is . . . if the 10K split was any indication, I have that 3:30 half in me somewhere. It's just, the weather wasn't on my side that day. It wasn't on the side of most of the other runners I know who were also out there on the course that day. Mother Nature had other plans for us. Today just wasn't our day.

The thing is . . . despite not actually beating my first half marathon time, I came close. I came really close, especially when you consider that weight I had regained since that race. I thought that extra weight slowed me down and it did, to a point, but this race just proved that size does not indicate speed or success.

Also, that first half marathon, the one I did for the 2013 Rock 'N' Roll Cleveland Half used a totally different route and when I ran the exact same Cleveland Half in 2014 it took me well over four hours, so in that regard this was a course PR and that *totally* counts.

17

Rita Hayworth, the Shawshank Redemption, and Me

Whenever I tell people I used to be a prison librarian, they always want to know if it's anything like *Orange Is the New Black* or *The Shawshank Redemption*. Obviously, working in a prison is an experience unto itself. So sprinkle a little bit of *Orange* here and a little *Shawshank* there and mix in some totally bizarre experiences that fall under "truth is stranger than fiction" and it was pretty much the most unique situation I've ever been in. Because I worked at an all-male facility, and given the heavy library focus, it was more Shawshank than anything else.

Adapted from the Stephen King novella *Rita Hayworth and the Shawshank Redemption,* the movie tells the story of Andy Dufresne, a Maine banker wrongfully convicted of the murder of his wife and her lover. He is sent to Shawshank State Penitentiary to serve his double life sentences and it is there that his life gets that chance for redemption. Seeing an opportunity, Andy takes on the role of expanding the prison library, which previously had consisted of a small cart pushed around by an older inmate named Brooks. Thanks to Andy's intervention, the library becomes a popular place among the prison population and inmates without a high school diploma are given alternative methods to graduate. Andy's own fate includes a well-executed narrow escape aided by a Hollywood starlet. (Without giving away too much, that's both a very literal and very figurative interpretation of what happens.)

In 1994, the novella was made into the Academy Award-nominated film starring Tim Robbins and Morgan Freeman. The film did horribly at the box office, but was redeemed (see what I did there?) thanks to video stores and cable television.

The Shawshank Redemption is one of my absolute favorite movies of all time, and it was long before I found myself behind bars. (Granted, y'know, I was there voluntarily—unlike the inmates I supervised in the prison library.) Like the Shawshank State Penitentiary, the library I managed was one of the more popular spots in the prison and was full to capacity every single day. Through the prison's education department, we also offered GED classes for those inmates who had previously dropped out of high school.

Along with being one of my favorite movies, *The Shawshank Redemption* is also one of my dad's favorite movies and was filmed in my home state at the Ohio State Reformatory down in Mansfield, Ohio. The city of Mansfield is located about eighty miles southwest of Cleveland, the halfway point between Lake Erie and our state capital Columbus. Mansfield is very proud of its Hollywood history, as is the entire county of Richland since many areas were also featured in this film and others. The opening scene of *The Shawshank Redemption,* with the double homicide that sets off the events in the movie, was filmed at Malabar Farms in nearby Lucas, Ohio. In May 1945,

Humphrey Bogart and Lauren Bacall exchanged wedding vows in the residential home on the property, known as the "Big House."

Tours are given at all of the major filming locations, including the Ohio State Reformatory, which hasn't housed inmates in its gothic walls since 1990; a few years ago the Shawshank Trail was established there. A self-paced driving tour, the Shawshank Trail allows film fans to travel the area by car and visit *Shawshank*'s fourteen filming locations.

In the summer of 2000, shortly before I started college, the official Shawshank Trail wasn't around yet, but my dad and I decided to do our own. We picked a Saturday afternoon and started planning out the places we wanted to try and visit.

All was well and good until about a week before our trip, when I tripped on a pair of shoes in our garage and managed to sprain my ankle. Because of course I would. We still made the trip down to Mansfield, only now I had an ankle wrapped in ACE Bandages and was on crutches.

So. You know. That was fun.

We didn't even get to see inside the prison that day, just kind of drove around scoping out some of the filming locations in the area.

Needless to say, a decade later, I was still anxious for my own Shawshank Redemption and while it took a while, as soon as I heard about the July 2015 inaugural Shawshank Hustle—an out-and-back 7K course that began and ended at the Ohio State Reformatory—I immediately told my dad about it and we agreed to sign up as soon as registration opened in January 2015. The fact that it was held in July, a month I still required a race to complete my racing goal, was an added bonus.

My dad had never run an official race. But he apparently doesn't mind the dreadmill and uses one at his gym when he goes to work out. But he was excited to run his first race not just with his daughter, but also with a theme focused on one of his favorite movies.

In the weeks prior to the event, the race committee sent out the usual race day information. Naturally, due to the location, there were some unusual informational pieces in the email, including the fact that parking at the former prison was going to be *extremely* limited. While the familiar and iconic Ohio State Reformatory is now a tourist attraction, there is still a very real operational prison right next door. Prisons, understandably, are highly guarded facilities. They don't take too well to weird, random people showing up and crowding around the yard. Even when I worked at a prison we had to keep our cars and plates on file. So strange cars using their parking lot? Ha, yeah, no. Not happening.

Instead, a large overflow parking lot a couple miles away was to be used on race day with buses transporting runners from the parking lot to the prison before the race.

As out-of-towners, this meant that packet pick-up was going to be, like, the worst thing ever, as this was a destination race and they had limited hours the night before the race.

Friday afternoon I left work and headed straight to my parents' house. After a brief visit with my mom, I threw my stuff in my dad's car and we hit the road. With a drive that was close to an hour and a half ahead of us, we opted for next-day packet pick-up.

It was dark by the time we got into the city limits, but my dad wanted to at least get a general sense of where our hotel was in relationship to the prison. Lights were on in the turrets and as we closed in on the compound, I caught my breath just driving past its beauty.

We then went to the hotel to check in and get settled. At this point we only had a couple of options, neither of them ideal: Option A was to wake up at 4:30 a.m., get ready, drive to the prison to get a good parking spot, get our packets and then just hang out in the car for four hours. Option B was to wake up at 4:30 a.m. drive to the prison, get our packets, then drive back to the hotel and sleep for another hour or two before getting up, getting ready, and driving to the overflow lot where we could use the bus service to get us back to the prison.

We decided to go with Option B.

So at 4:30 a.m., after what felt like only an hour after I went to bed, the alarm on my phone went off and I stumbled out of the bed. My dad was sleeping on the couch, but my fumbling around in the dark roused him awake. We pulled ourselves together enough to hop into the car and drove over.

Prisons are unique institutions. There really is nothing quite like them, and I'd prefer people just trust me on this rather than set some goal to find out for themselves. (Unless, of course, a librarian reading this is interested in a highly rewarding nontraditional career path.)

While the historic Ohio State Reformatory is not an operational prison, because of its close proximity to the very operational Richland

Correctional Institution, there are still guards that patrol the grounds and they don't allow strangers to just walk up to the building. Even if they did, they aren't going to let them do it at 4:30 a.m. when it's pitch black out.

On top of that, while the Ohio State Reformatory may not function as a prison these days, it comes with a long history and the preservation society in charge of its care hosts tours and events throughout the year to maintain the upkeep costs. Because of its historic and supposedly haunted history, they also offer overnight ghost hunts and multiple paranormal television shows have visited the site. Every October they also turn the prison into an intense haunted house and several of my prison coworkers made it an annual autumn trip. Surprisingly, given my love for Halloween, I never went. I like haunted houses but the word on the street was this one really goes above and beyond. The normal baseline for haunted houses is enough for me, *thankyouverymuch*. No above nor beyond needed. Plus, given the institution's reputation for being legitimately haunted, and being someone who believes in all of that mumbo jumbo, it seemed a little like tempting fate.

One of these overnight ghost-hunting visits was leaving the prison as we arrived. I told my Dad he could wait in the car and I'd go pick our packets up. This, after all, was not my first time at the (racing) rodeo.

I've had the opportunity to run in several inaugural races: the Rock 'N' Roll Cleveland Half Marathon, the Christmas Story 10K, and the Shawshank Hustle. With any new venture there are always going to be some kinks that need to be worked out. Add in a popular film with a cult following and a prison location, and the number of kinks seem to exponentially grow.

For one thing, there seemed to be limited communication between the racing organization and the Ohio State Reformatory. Because while we were told packet pick-up would start at 5 a.m., those of who arrived at that time were made to stand outside the closed prison gates until close to 5:30 a.m., because we had to wait until all of the ghost hunters had left. Honestly, the guards that were on duty didn't really seem to know what to do with those of us waiting, and it seemed as if they weren't quite sure why we were there, but finally the gates opened and we were allowed in.

Just thinking about walking up that long, dark driveway towards the prison still gives me goosebumps. Because while I was looking at the historic Ohio State Reformatory, what I *saw* was the Shawshank State Penitentiary. With its grand front entrance and turret rising high, it looked less like a prison and more like a fortress. A majestic, beautiful, magnificent fortress.

I was grinning like a silly fan girl when I walked into the white tent to pick up our packets (which included a GLOW IN THE DARK SHIRT). Once I had those, I jumped back in the car and we returned to the hotel. The first thing I had to do was check out if the shirt really glowed in the dark, so I locked myself in the bathroom with the lights off and grinned when the greenish glow was reflected in the mirror.

After grabbing a short nap back at the hotel, we got dressed into our running outfits. On the drive over I realized that when I picked up our packets I forgot to pick up the very necessary safety pins to affix the bibs to our shirts, so I suggested he just drop me off then head to the overflow lot and I'd wait for him at the bus drop-off spot.

This is where things got . . . complicated, because being that this was an inaugural race, the racing committee *way* underestimated the amount of buses needed to transport everyone from the overflow lot. They had also underestimated the amount of family and spectators who would arrive and want to hang out at the prison, just because. Not that I can really blame them: this is a tourist destination on its own. But how many people think to just go on a random weekend?

Dad dropped me off at 7:30 a.m. The race was supposed to start at 8:30 a.m. but due to so many people still waiting back at the overflow lot they kept pushing the time back, first to 8:45 a.m., then to 9 a.m. I waited anxiously on the sidewalk by the buses, worried I'd somehow missed him in the crowd of people and he was waiting somewhere else looking for me. Then, right after the race finally started, I saw him climbing off one of the bright yellow school busses. Luckily, because there were so many people and because we'd be in the back anyway because of our speed, we managed to make it in the starting line right when we needed to.

The course took us up through the parking lot of the Ohio State Reformatory, and out onto the street. In other races I've run, the race is able to have entire streets closed down for at least the beginning part of the race. In this case, only one side of the road was available to runners, which meant there were 3,000 people bottlenecking their way down the street for a quarter of a mile. We were so cramped that running was impossible and as we slowly walked, my dad turned to me and said he hoped it wasn't like this the whole course.

Once the main road turned, the other side of the street was open to us and we were able to spread out. I started doing my run-walk-run intervals while my dad "jogged" beside me.

That was his word. Jog. It's a weighted word, jogging, fraught with lots of emotions. I would say that he ran because to me—and I'm sure to others as well—anything above a walk counts as running. But if he wants to say he jogged, I'll let him say he jogged. He also broke it down for me, the differences between walking, jogging, and running. It had something to do with feet. Like how many feet are on the ground at any one time. I think he also may have used horses as an example. So based on this information he'd read somewhere the placement of his feet meant he was jogging.

But, whatever. He was totally running.

Now filming for *The Shawshank Redemption* took place all over the city of Mansfield and so our course took us right into the quaint downtown with its green square and white gazebo. On that small patch of grass was a bench marked Brooks's Bench and the exterior of other buildings were highlighted with signs and also large cutouts of Tim Robbins and Morgan Freeman, meant for photo opportunities.

A few weeks before the race, I ordered a custom shirt that I still wear at every race. It's bright blue with a winged shoe on the front. On the back it says *It's not last place, it's running with police escort.*

At the time, my friend Andrew asked why I would put it on the back of the shirt, when nobody would see it. I told him that the people behind me would. The back of the pack would. Those were the people I wanted to see it, the ones who are slow, the ones who are in last place.

The Shawshank Hustle was the first time I wore it for a race, and I wasn't sure what the reaction would be. But several times while running, I had people from the back pass me and compliment me on my shirt. Ironically, because this was one of those novelty themed races, it attracted thousands of people, not all of them runners and our pace kept us firmly planted in the middle of the pack.

We were also firmly planted at the height of high summer and running in a rather hilly city. Everyone around us was drenched in sweat and feeling the heat and humidity. Since the race also started late, we were out there running slightly later in the day than originally planned.

As we climbed the final hill, the course turned left back onto the main road. Soon the prison was back within our sights. Against the backdrop of the bright blue sky and lush green grass, I could see what attracted the filmmakers when they were scouting locations.

We ran down the parking lot and entrance and towards the prison. The finish line was at the end of the large paved entrance and as we ran towards it, the prison grew larger until we were practically right at its front door.

In terms of goodies: the shirts, the finisher's medals, which also glowed in the dark, and our race entry also provided us with an opportunity to tour the prison for free. (Well done, race organizers. Well done.) It was so hot and the line was so long, we decided to skip it and just head home. First, however, this meant waiting for the buses to return to take us to the overflow lot. Thankfully they seemed a little more organized after the race.

We stood in the parking lot with the other runners, waiting for the buses to return. The sun rose high overhead and as we waited, the heat started to catch up with me. Even with sunglasses, the sun hurt my eyes to the point of needing to keep them closed and I started to feel really lightheaded. Going over my food and drink options that morning, I realized this is what dehydration probably feels like.

Fuck. I think I'm going to pass out.

On my left was my dad, trying to engage me in conversation. I nodded politely, giving halfhearted responses in an attempt to appear like I was paying attention. All the while, though, I was scoping out the scene. The parking lot was crowded with cars and the surface was covered in rocks. If I *did* pass out, I'd mostly likely hit my head on a fender or slam it down into a nice hard pillow of stones. Neither of those prospects were appealing. Every couple of seconds I'd turn towards the main road hoping to see the buses. I didn't even need all of them, just one. Just one little bus that would get me away from the hot sun.

Fuck, fuck, fuck. Breathe. Just breathe.

I bent over at the waist, hands on my hips.

Unaware of what was physically and mentally going on inside of my head, my dad was trying to keep up a continuing conversation that I was only half-listening to and not at all participating in. Finally, I turned to him and politely, but firmly, asked if he would please stop talking for just a few minutes.

"Are you okay?"

"I will be, I just need a couple of minutes."

He nodded and offered me the rest of the water left in the plastic bottle he'd picked up at the finish line. I'd already finished mine and happily finished off his, too.

Finally, after what felt like forever, the buses arrived. We climbed on board and I started to feel better as soon as I sat down. There wasn't any air conditioning, but the windows were open and a nice breeze blew through, providing relief.

The bus dropped us off at the overflow lot and we walked over to where Dad had parked several hours before. We got in, he cranked up the AC, and we headed home.

The Shawshank Hustle was my dad's first official race. It was my twenty-sixth. I was also now over halfway done with my 2015 race goal.

By now, I'd been running for over three and a half years, a fact I still had a hard time wrapping my head around. I had originally started running to lose weight and while I was successful at the start, I was not quite so successful in recent months. But despite that, despite my size, and the number on the scale, I'd completed dozens of 5Ks, multiple 10Ks, and three half marathons.

What would have happened had I not heeded that original email my sister sent me, expressing concern for my health? Where would I be? *Would* I still be?

Oh, sure. Some of the time, it sucked. Running is fucking hard. Not all runs are wonderful; some are downright awful and make me want to quit running altogether. But then I have runs like this one, where I get to spend a weekend with my dad, have a small road trip, get one step closer to my 2015 running goal, log some miles, *and* visit the setting of one of my favorite films based on a book by one of my favorite authors. Well, I guess it's like Stephen King wrote: *It always comes down to just two choices. Get busy living or get busy dying.*

18
The Tortoise
and the Hares

An unexpected benefit to being named an Ambassador for the 2015 Cleveland Half Marathon was that it gave me the opportunity to connect with some amazing other runners. And by "amazing" I mean fast. And by "fast" I mean these are individuals who are literally twice as fast as I am: in the 3 hours and 46 minutes it took me to run 13.1 miles in 2015, these speed demons were finishing up 26.2.

One in particular had her eye on the big prize. In the short time that I had come to know Jamie, I had quickly become inspired by her story. Like me, Jamie had once weighed over 300 pounds and had lost a significant amount of weight. Unlike me, Jamie has managed to keep it all off all these years later. She's also a beast and had set her sights on Boston. Her qualifying race would (hopefully) be the 2015 Akron Marathon, held in September.

Those of us who know her—and especially those of us who have run and trained alongside her—wanted to be there for Jamie when she crossed the finish line. Some of the other Ambassadors were also running either the Akron Half or Full and we realized this would be a perfect opportunity for a Family Reunion of sorts. Unfortunately, not all of us were in a position to sign up for any of the big races. We either didn't have the time to train, or were training for another long distance race after Akron, or we just didn't have the funds.

It was Andrew who first presented the idea of a relay team. Akron, like many cities, offers the Marathon option as a team activity. In this case, five people take turns each running a specific section, or leg, of the full distance. Your final time is a group effort and your place depends entirely on how fast (or slow) your other teammates are.

When the idea of a Relay Team was first brought up, it was the height of summer and I was in the process of mapping out my races for the second half of the year. In January, I had committed to my 2015 racing goal, and as rates are cheaper the further out you sign up, registering months in advance was always a good idea. September was a month I was struggling with to find a race that fit my schedule, so when a call went out into the group to see if anyone would be interested in doing the relay, I immediately indicated my interest.

Going in, my team was fully aware of the fact that I am nowhere near as fast as them. In fact, I'm downright slow. During the winter and spring months, as we followed each other's training progress for Cleveland, they knew that I was hoping to run a 3:30 half, a sluggish pace for these speed demons. I felt it necessary to reiterate to them that I'm slow. Not in a self-deprecating kind of way; just in a matter-of-fact kind of way.

For Akron, I'd be running the fourth leg of our relay, which was 3.6 miles, a distance that at this point I felt fairly comfortable with; so, my training was halfhearted and haphazard at best. It was also summer, which meant that the heat and humidity contributed to this slow runner running even more slowly than usual. My running related social media posts increased as I lamented 17- and 18-minute miles. I've never been embarrassed by my speed, but I also didn't want to be in a position where I felt like I was holding the rest of the group back. Race days can be unpredictable and while I tend to run faster during a race than I do during training, if experience has taught me anything, it's that shit happens out on the course. I could have trained with the best of them and been at the top of my game, but come race day there was no way of knowing if I'd get injured, or if Mother Nature would decide to wreak havoc. So my decision to post my slower times wasn't about looking for validation or encouragement from fellower runners; it was more about making sure, really making sure, that my team knew exactly what they had signed up for when they asked me to to join them.

As far as marathons go, Akron is still a relative baby, with its inaugural event dating only to 2003 (versus nearby Cleveland, which will be celebrating its fortieth year in 2017). That said, in its relatively short lifespan, Akron has grown from a local race with 3,775 participants to a national sporting event with tens of thousands of runners descending on Northeast Ohio each year.

While the half marathon distance wasn't added until 2007, there has always been some form of a relay at Akron. In 2003 and 2004, the race hosted the North American Men's Marathon Relay Championships, as well as the USA Track & Field National Club Marathon Relay Championships. The relay got so large that it sold out in 2009, and in 2011 it was ranked as the largest United States marathon relay by Running USA.

Akron is also one of the few marathons that continues to employ a blue line painted on the street to mark the course. The race organizers take their blue line seriously, branding it on everything from swag, to the floor of the Expo, to even locally made doughnuts with blue stripes of frosting. Needless to say, running the Blue Line endears runners and gives those that finish a sense of pride they don't always get at other races.

The week leading up to the race I was fighting off a cold, which is never fun, especially when you have an impending race. I've raced sick before and really didn't want to have to do it again, especially when there were other people counting on me. Luckily my manager knew about the race, so when I asked to take a sick day that Friday in order to give my body time to rest, she was totally on board.

Not working the day before the race not only gave me a chance to take it easy, but it also meant I got to pick up my packet earlier than originally planned along with a new pair of running shoes at the Expo. Downtown Akron was buzzing with that infectious energy that all runners carry with them in the hours before a race. The city and the Expo in particular, was electric with it.

I knew that the other Cleveland Ambassadors running on Saturday would be floating in and out of the Expo at some point during the day, but I only managed to cross paths with Andrew. It had been months since we'd seen each other in person and, even then, we'd only met maybe twice before. But running always brings about this intuitive sense of camaraderie and connection. So few people do what we do, that when you find another person who shares a similar level of passion you instantly bond and things like time and distance lose all meaning.

After getting all of my race day items and information, I headed to my parents' house, where I was spending the night, since they live far closer to Akron than I do. I was still going to have to wake up ridiculously early on Saturday morning, but not as early as I would have had I stayed at my place. I was super excited about my new shoes, but also knew it would be a bad, bad idea to wear them race day. However, I did go for a short one-mile run before dinner to try them out and to give my legs one final workout before the race. Then it was an early bedtime, as I had a 5 a.m. wake-up call and had to be on the road to Akron by 5:45 a.m.

Running races in cities other than Cleveland always leaves me feeling super nervous, mostly for logistical reasons. When I'm in Cleveland, I know where to park and how much time I need to give myself to get to the start line. In unfamiliar cities I tend to overcompensate and arrive way earlier than necessary. (To be fair, I tend to arrive *everywhere* way earlier than necessary. I'm one of those really obnoxious "being on time is late" people.) But with a race as big as Akron, that works out in my favor as I was able to quickly find convenient parking. After making sure I had all of my gear, I locked up the car and headed towards the start line. Of course, it was dark and I had no idea where I was going but, again, with a race as big as Akron it was easy to just follow the crowd and, eventually, follow the sounds.

My team had made tentative plans to meet before the race and we were all attempting to text each other to try and figure out where everyone was located at the start. Naturally we weren't the only Relay Team trying to coordinate and the cell phone lines were jammed, taking messages forever to get through. Finally, I located most of my team with the exception of our fearless leader and first-leg runner, Andrew, who was still missing in action. We knew he was somewhere in the crowd and working on getting to the corral before the start, but we weren't able to see him before the race started. Instead, we stood on the sidelines and cheered on all the runners as the race started.

Melissa was Leg 2 and could walk to her starting point and since Andrew had told her that he'd only need about 40 minutes, she quickly hurried off after we saw all the runners cross the start line to find where she needed to be. Another team member, Stephanie, could also walk to her starting point, while the final two leg-runners, Dan and I, had to take shuttle buses to our respective exchange spots. Being that it was a relay, however, we all had plenty of time, so Dan and I walked Stephanie to her spot before we went looking for the shuttles.

When we first decided to do the relay, we didn't put much thought into who would run which section. It was only after all signing up that we started divvying up each leg. Knowing that it was going to take me longer to run my distance no matter what, I planned on volunteering to take the shortest leg, which was 3.6 miles, so when Andrew preemptively asked if I'd be okay running that one, I said yes right away. My other team members would all be running distances closer to 6 miles, yet they'd all be finishing their legs in a shorter period of time than my goal of an hour.

I was reminded of this fact while sitting on the shuttle bus where all of the Leg 4 participants were chatting as we made our way along the streets of Akron. Across the aisle from me was a small group of women making conversation and one in particular caught my attention. She was probably in her mid-twenties and looked like someone I would consider a "traditional" runner. That is, if she were to casually mention to a stranger that she runs, said stranger would not give her the incredulous and/or surprised look that I often get. As much as I like to believe I got my 13.1 tattoo for myself, I think a part of me got it for other people. It's a permanent flag to wave that indicates my membership in the running community.

So this woman was talking about how while she was training, her team hadn't yet decided who would be doing which leg, but as soon as she mentioned that she was running something close to 14-minute miles, her team members straight up told her that she'd be running the short leg. Based on the look she wore while communicating this story, I could tell how much it hurt her to have these people she considered friends judge her for being a slow runner. Here I was with my 16-minute miles, proud of having gotten those down from 17- or 18-minute miles, running on a team with members who run 7- and 8-minute miles. It would have been very easy, even understandable, if they decided they didn't want me on their team because they had a time goal they wanted to meet and I would hold them back. But they didn't do that. Those hares welcomed this tortoise with open arms and I have no doubt that if a couple months before when Andrew asked if I'd be okay running the shortest leg, I had spoken up and said that no, I'd prefer doing one of the longer ones, they would have completely supported that, even if it meant our overall time would be even slower.

I find myself apologizing for my speed a lot, often when I don't actually need to. Or feeling like I need to explain or justify it. But my team didn't care about my speed, they didn't care if they had a slow runner on the team. All they cared about was having ME on the team, regardless of pace or place. I already knew I was running with the best damn team out there, but listening to that woman talk about her own team made me realize that the individual people who made up my team were all pretty damn awesome as well.

When the bus stopped at the exchange point, one of the volunteers got on board to go over some final instructions relating specifically to the relay. Each team member wore the same bib number as his or her other members and we would line up along the street and wait for the announcer to call out our bib number as our teammate came running up around the corner. Posts with bib numbers in chronological order had been put up and we were supposed to stay as close in order as possible and meet our teammate in the street by our number.

I got to the exchange with about an hour to wait, but I happened to have two friends also running Leg 4, including Megan. This is the same Megan who several years before had waited around an extra twenty minutes or so at the finish line of my very first race, just so she could see me cross it. Because the Cleveland running community is pretty small, we often run into each other at races. While we were waiting for our numbers to be called, we stood around chatting and catching up. She knew I had set a goal of running one race a month and asked how my progress was going and what races I planned on doing for the remaining months of the year.

The marathon relay follows the same course as the full marathon, which meant that along with cheering on the other Leg 4 Relay runners, we got to first cheer on the elite runners as they passed by us. Whether you are fast or slow, hell, whether or not you even run, it's impossible to look at the elites and not be blown away by the level of athleticism visible in every muscle of their body. Their dedication to the sport can't be ignored and watching them in action is absolutely awe-inspiring.

Soon, the Leg 3 runners started making their way up the hill. Slow and sporadic at first, they quickly began to gain momentum and it became even more important to pay attention to the numbers being called out. Before the race, we had all given our team an idea of how long it would take each person to complete their section, so I knew when to anticipate Stephanie and sure enough, she was right on schedule. When I heard our number called, I stepped out into the road, and as soon as Stephanie and I made eye contact we both kind of did a little jump of excitement. She handed me the blue slap bracelet (I told you Akron took their blue line branding seriously!) and I was off.

During my training I had been experimenting with my run-walk-run intervals by doing 30 seconds of running, followed by 30 seconds of walking. I had seen some success with this timing so for race day I decided to go with what had been working and right from the very beginning I felt strong and confident and knew I had a very good chance of beating my goal of one hour. I went in my mental zone and followed that famous blue line.

I started at Mile Seventeen and, thanks to the prior work of my teammates, I found myself for the first time ever in the front of the pack. Considering I will probably NEVER EVER IN A MILLION YEARS experience the front of the pack again, I mentally soaked in every single step of my 3.6 miles, watching in awe as the runners passed me. Following good race etiquette, I stayed to the side of the course and out of the way of more speedy roadsters. While it was probably pretty obvious that I was a bit out of my element, that sense of cama-raderie came through from those around me and a couple of the runners passed me with encouraging words.

Halfway between Miles Eighteen and Nineteen, I saw a flash of pink out of the corner of my eye and as the runner came up from behind me with a wave, I realized it was fellow Cleveland Marathon Ambassador Jamie. She, along with the other Ambassadors, was one of the reasons I was out there that day. These Ambassadors made me feel like I had found my running family, so getting to be the one that saw her on the course meant the world to me and made me realize how grateful I am to be a part of this amazing and supportive group of athletes.

After I passed the marker for Mile Twenty, I knew I only had about a half mile to go, so I just kept my pace and headed towards the exchange zone for the fifth leg. When Dan saw me rounding the corner, he waved and I waved back. That gave me the push to pick up my pace for the final tenth of a mile and I handed him the bracelet and watched him go.

My leg ended in a park and as I made my way across the grass to catch the shuttle which would take me to the finish line, I texted my team to let them know that Dan was headed home.

The Akron races finish on the field of Canal Park, home of the local minor league baseball stadium. Runners enter from the back, essen-tially the outfield, and basically run along the first baseline, ending near home plate. The rest of the field is transformed into the Finisher Festival, where relay team members can meet up after finishing and take advantage of the free beer and food before finding any family members who were waiting and watching in the stands. It still is the most amazing finish line I've yet seen and I was, in the words of the infamous Scarlett O'Hara, "pea-green with envy" seeing Dan get to run it.

I made it to the stadium and found my team minutes after Jamie finished, but I was there in time to see Dan come down the final stretch of his leg and cross the finish line at 3:57:59. My personal time for my section was 57:36, which put me below the hour goal I had. At 16-minute miles I was quite satisfied with my finish, especially considering the numbers I had been showing while training.

In the Aesop's immortal tale, a hare's hubris is his downfall, when the slow and steady tortoise sneaks past him. What the fable assumes is that unequal partners are fundamentally at odds with each other. That the slower half of a pair somehow can't run—let alone finish—the race with their faster counterpart because of unequal speeds or abilities. I have no doubt that in some instances that very well may be the case. I, however, have always been lucky enough to defy that stereotype. Take, for instance, the runners in the front of the pack who encouraged me along the course. Those words of support weren't unique—it happens at almost every race I run. Because we know that despite the guise of it being a race and there being a first place and a last place, ultimately we aren't running against each other; we are running *with* each other. This occurs all the time: it happens when I'm out doing a training run, pounding the streets of Cleveland, and another runner and I exchange nods. It happens when a coworker sees my half marathon tattoo and we start discussing various races we've run or ones that are upcoming.

And it happened that day in September when a handful of hares helped this slow and steady runner do the impossible: run a sub–4-hour marathon.

19
Finding My Voice

The Shawshank Hustle and Akron Marathon Relay fell in the middle of an otherwise very busy summer, and satisfied two of my required monthly races. In June, I had run the Nature's Bin 5K, with my boyfriend Ben joining me. Ben doesn't run a lot of organized races, but we thought it would be fun to do one together. And by "together" I mean we started at the start line standing next to each other and I met him at the finish line. He's faster than me, but not by too much, and it was fun spending the whole race with the view of his bright yellow shirt just a little bit ahead of me. In August, I ran the Rock City 5K, an inaugural race that had an accompanying half marathon. With the time of year and rock 'n' roll theme, I think it was attempting to replace the canceled Run Rock 'N' Roll Half.

That same summer I also launched my "Running with a Police Escort" podcast.

Running can be a very lonely sport sometimes. Granted, that's sometimes my own fault, as I prefer to run alone. But I very rarely actually feel alone when that happens, even when I'm in the very back and/or last place and haven't seen another runner for miles.

It's only after the race, after crossing that finish line that I start to wish I had other people to talk to about the experiences of being in the back of the pack. All of my local running friends are fast and therefore have a much different perception of racing than I do, which is fine, but it can sometimes make me feel like my experiences are solitary ones. But I know that's not true, though—I know that the obstacles and challenges I've faced happen to other slow runners all over the place. The key was figuring out a way to talk to other slow runners.

The idea for the podcast came from one of the online running groups I belong to. That February, after the SnoBall 5K, I was talking to some fellow runners about having been last and having the police car behind me. Someone commented that she always thought it would be fun to have a podcast for last-place finishers called DNF: *dead fucking last.*

Since she didn't actually have any desire to make such a podcast, I asked if she minded if I borrowed the idea. She said it was fine. I also decided to put a slightly more positive spin on the title. Being last isn't necessarily a bad thing what with that whole police escort thing happening and all.

I had no experience with podcasting aside from being a listener, but really, how hard could it be? So I started doing research. Lots of research. Hours and months of research. Research about equipment and recording and hosting and getting it on iTunes and it turns out podcasting is slightly more complicated than I realized.

I mean, it's not SUPER complicated. It's not like rocket science that requires assistance from Neil deGrasse Tyson. But, y'know, it's still work. There's a lot that needs to be done. It's also not free—it can be done on the cheap, even the very cheap, but at the very least, most hosting services (that thing that lets a podcast be uploaded to iTunes) require a monthly fee.

Between that, building a website, and not wanting to cheap out on microphones and equipment, I decided to give crowdsourcing a try. I was hoping that the theme of the podcast would be enough to maybe encourage some people to back the project on Kickstarter. If not, well, I'd figure out a way to pay for it all myself.

I sort of underestimated just how much support there would be for this endeavor, because not only did I hit my goal within the first 24 hours, by the end of the campaign I had doubled it.

Granted, I crunched some numbers and was aiming for the absolute bare minimum it would take to finance the podcast for a year, so I was only asking for a couple hundred of dollars initially. But still. These people, friends, family, and even some strangers, gave freely of their own money to support my podcast.

My first few guests were cultivated from my personal group of running friends and in the summer of 2015, I went live.

A couple of weeks later I flew to Denver to attend the FitBloggin 2015 conference, where I got up in front of the entire conference and presented on being a slow runner. The response was overwhelming—turns out, there are a lot of slow runners out there and they, like me, want their voices heard and their stories told.

Summer was winding down, the leaves changing from the bright green of summer to the burning oranges and reds of autumn. There's nothing I love more than that first fall run, with the air crisp and cool, as leaves snap and crack under my shoes. The change in season also meant daylight hours were getting shorter, limiting my running time in the sun.

October brought the Great Beer Chase 5K. Hosted by Cleveland's own Great Lakes Brewing Company and timed to align with Beer Week, the Great Beer Chase was a 5K that ran through the Ohio City neighborhood of Cleveland, home of Great Lakes Brewing. Sometimes races get names that don't have much meaning, but in this case, there literally was beer to chase. Or, well, runners dressed to represent different GLBC brews including Burning River, Eliot Ness, and Commodore Perry (that last one took me a minute to figure out when I saw him on the course).

The race was a simple out-and-back. It started at the brewery, ran about a mile and a half, then turned around and came back. During the whole race, I stuck to my run-walk-run intervals. Ahead of me, keeping a fast walking pace, was a woman in black. She spent the whole race walking. That is, she spent the whole race walking up until the moment about two miles in that I passed her.

When running with intervals, I tend to keep a consistent pace and eventually I often will get enough of a lead to pass people who had spent the first part of the race ahead of me. That scenario happened here and as soon as I passed her, she started to run. This was the first time for the entire race that she ran, so I can hardly think it's a coincidence. She'd pull ahead enough to pass me then start walking again but as soon as I passed her, she'd start running again.

I wasn't offended. In fact, I found it funny more than anything else. I mean, if she needs me to motivate her to run then, well, I'll play my part. But I made her *work* for that finish, believe you me. When we got closer to the finish I fucking booked it to that finish line, running as fast as I absolutely could.

Don't hate the player, hate the game.

Great Lakes Brewing Company had fun with this one. Not only was there beer at the end, but, our race medals were branded bottle openers on a ribbon.

Cleveland, I love you.

Like many cities, Cleveland hosts a Turkey Trot every Thanksgiving morning, offering both a 5K and a 5 Mile race. In 2015, I was scheduled to run the Christmas Story 10K in early December, so the 5 Mile distance fit into my race training perfectly. (Might as well also take advantage of an opportunity to burn off some calories in anticipation of all the pumpkin pie later in the day.)

Unfortunately, the night before I started having some stomach issues that left me feeling all kinds of icky. But, it was the very end of November—if I didn't run this race, I wasn't going to have another opportunity to race this month and I couldn't come so close to finishing my goal and failing in the second-to-last month.

The gun was set to go off at 9:30 a.m. and the course was going to be open for two hours after that. Even if I really wasn't feeling well and decided to walk the entire 5 miles, and even if there were a bunch of other runners, I should still be well ahead of that course closure.

In theory.

In actuality, the race started fifteen minutes late. There we were, all 3,000 runners, warmed up and ready to go, anxiously biding our time on Lakeside Avenue. The weather was on our side and it wasn't as snowy and cold as prior Turkey Trots had been, but even then I still kept checking my watch every few minutes, impatient to start.

Then, because there were so many runners, and because I was observing the proper race etiquette and situated myself in the back, it took me ten minutes to get to the start line. Add to that the fact that I hadn't been feeling well that week, so had to walk more than I planned . . . my pace was behind what I had hoped.

But the real problem was that while the race started late, they—be it the race committee or the city of Cleveland or both—failed to adjust the rest of the schedule and push back the course closure time. Suddenly, I had lost half an hour of viable, necessary running time on an open course before I even started.

Of course, I had no way of knowing that at the time. All I could do was do my intervals and try to keep up my pace as long as I could.

I've run this race before in freezing cold and snow. This time around, it was slightly chilly, but the sky was bright blue with few clouds. For a race in late November, there really wasn't any better weather.

My intervals kept me going for the first two miles, but after that my stomach started to feel icky again and I had to switch to straight walking. I walked my second and third miles, through the quiet streets of Cleveland, then at the start of the last mile, I began to do my intervals again.

This was a race that actually had a pretty substantial back of the pack. There was a pocket of us who had been keeping a relatively consistent pace together for the whole race and we were all eager to get to the finish line. The only problem was that we had no idea where we were going. With other races that have lots of turns there are usually little orange cones set up on corners with arrows pointing the course out to runners. If they had been up earlier, then they had already been taken down by the time we got back, and the policemen and guards who, no doubt, had spent the better part of the morning directing the faster runners to the correct turns to end up at the finish, were now busy directing all of the cars moving through the downtown city streets of Cleveland. One of our group had to go so far *as to ask another runner who had already finished* where we were supposed to turn to get back.

Turning that last corner, I stopped short.

Just a couple hours ago, this place was full of people and sponsors and spectators. It was a ghost town at this point. All barriers had been taken down and the post-race food, drinks, and sponsors had fled. There was nothing, save the blue finish mat and a couple of people from the race committee.

I paid my registration fee. I showed up. I ran my five miles. And I don't even get a damn banana for my effort?

ARE YOU FUCKING KIDDING ME?!?

I don't begrudge the race or city for being unable to keep a course open indefinitely for those of us in the back of the pack, but when I go out of my way to check course times and only register for races where I feel confident I'll be able to finish, I do so with the expectation that a race will either (a) start on time or (b) push back the course closure if it starts late. By doing neither of those things, the only people punished are the slow runners who are the very runners that need all the time the race offers.

And I wasn't even in last place; there were still a couple of people behind me. I have no idea what sort of finish line they encountered.

I don't think race committees do this on purpose, but sometimes it makes me feel like races aren't for me because I'm not fast. It's like myself, and other slow runners like me, are afterthoughts. Or, not even after thoughts because that assumes they are thinking about us at all—it's like we're lucky enough to just happen to get whatever's left over from the race after the fast runners finish.

It's not all organizations: I've run some races that treat last place just as well as first. But other times, I feel . . . forgotten.

Nobody puts Baby in a corner, dammit.

The back of the pack runners are "real runners," we just run a little slower than our fast counterparts and—as long as we stick to the course time limits—we deserve as much support and encouragement as the front of the pack. That, right there, is what pissed me off the most about the 2015 Turkey Trot: *I* stuck to the course time limits. *They* didn't. But I was the one who paid the price.

A week later I ran the Christmas Story 10K. It was the race's third year: I ran the first race in 2013, but had skipped the second, mostly because I was so totally not impressed with the medal.

No shame.

But this year, the theme was "Pink Nightmare" and the finisher's medal showed a little boy dressed in a pink bunny suit running with some leg lamps.

HERE. TAKE MY MONEY. PLEASE GIVE ME A PRETTY PINK MEDAL.

In 2013, I finished in 1:37:23. In 2015, about forty pounds heavier, I finished in 1:37:58.

Well, damn. I guess you really *can't* determine speed or success based on what a person looks like.

As I crossed that finish line and the volunteer put that medal around my neck, I had officially completed the goal I set out to achieve twelve months ago.

And as proud as I was of that, this was just one year, one goal. January 2016 was right around the corner and there were still lots of races to run.

But it was also December. Winter was coming, and I still had one more dragon to slay.

20

How I Learned to Stop Worrying and Love the Dreadmill

Cleveland really does have a thing for lovable losers because this slow runner was asked to come back as an Ambassador for the 2016 Cleveland Marathon races. I weighed the option of running the half for a third year in a row, but I also had to weigh the likelihood of me finally getting that PR against those final four miles. Neither the 2014 nor the 2015 race was particularly kind to me, and I'm not sure I was physically, emotionally, or mentally ready to come so close, only to be crushed by the last couple of miles yet again.

Then there was the fact that I was still so jealous of Dan, the final leg in our relay back in September, getting to cross that finish line in Canal Park and wanting that for myself. The Akron races are at the end of September, putting it seasonally closer to my very first half versus Cleveland's May schedule. Picking another fall race might just be what I needed to finally get that PR, so as soon as registration opened in early January, I signed up and got the Early Bird pricing. #winning.

(Of course, a couple of weeks later I found out that Stephen King would be appearing at the National Book Festival in Washington D.C. that very same weekend. Akron doesn't allow transfers, deferments, or refunds and I didn't buy the insurance because I'm an idiot who never buys the insurance. This would be my luck. But my desire to cross that finish line in Canal Park beat out even my love of Stephen King.)

But that meant I still had to pick my race for Cleveland's 2016 events. This year they introduced something new: a Challenge Series.

Traditionally for Cleveland Marathon Weekend, there is a 5K on a Saturday with the 10K, half, and full marathons on Sunday. Opting to make it more of a weekend event, the organization created some pairings and also included a brand-new 8K race on Saturday morning. If a runner signed up for one of the three Challenge Series options— 5K/10K, 8K/half, 8K/full—they'd get extra bling and some additional swag in their packet. Any of the distances could be run singularly as well, but this was just an added incentive.

Being that I love me some extra bling, I opted for the 5K/10K Challenge. The training wouldn't be as time-consuming as, say, a half marathon, but I would have to work on more back-to-back runs and getting used to going out there on tired legs.

This also meant that when training started in early February, it was still too cold and dark outside in the mornings to run outdoors before work.

This meant I only had one option.

I stepped on the treadmill, spreading my legs apart to put my feet on the sides while I got everything set up. My water bottle went in the cup holder on the right while my phone went in the cup holder on the left. In the middle of the dashboard I put my tablet.

This morning I was trying something new.

All the time I see friends post on social media about doing their long runs indoors. I'm talking eight, nine, sometimes even upwards of fifteen, sixteen miles on the *treadmill*. That's it, just running on the treadmill for distances equal to or greater than a half-fucking-marathon. Round and round the belt goes for several hours while you stare at a wall or out a window, if you're lucky. Just running along on a *treadmill*.

Like, *I literally cannot even.* (So much so I just keep putting it in italics because that is the only way I can reasonably express my complete and utter shock at this.)

Of course, when it's a fast runner we're talking only needing maybe a couple of hours out of the day to knock out a decent set of miles. Even if they're going to be running a five- or six-hour marathon on race day, most training plans stop a few miles short of the final distance, so they won't need that long on even their longest training run.

Which is exactly why I will never run a marathon. Well, six other reasons as well. Seven hours in total. Based on my half marathon PR, it would take me *at least* seven hours to complete a full marathon. Which is a problem since many marathon racing organizations cut off the course time at seven hours and my saying it would take me at least that long is probably being far too generous in my own abilities. It would probably take me closer to seven and a half hours, maybe eight depending on weather, course, how my training went, etc.

There are certain things I love enough to dedicate eight hours of my life to complete. These include marathon reading the brand-new book by a favorite author, and marathon watching the latest season of *Orange is the New Black* the day Netflix releases it. (Which, conveniently, started back up the weekend after I handed in the first draft of this book to my editor. Coincidence? I think not. Instead, it's almost like Netflix was rewarding me for all my hard work.)

But marathon *running* for eight hours?

Hahahahahahaha.

So, yeah, while I'm perfectly happy being someone who has completed multiple half marathons, there is no way I will ever, under any circumstances, run a full marathon. I'm not saying that to be flippant or facetious or to have someone come and tell me that I could totally do it.

Could I? Sure. Probably. It's like anything else, it's all a matter of how well I train. But do I want to? Hell no. I have a limit on the tread-mill. I can only go so long before dying of complete and utter boredom. This is usually in the realm of about five minutes, which, obviously, isn't ideal for someone training for races while living in a city where the treadmill is a necessity at certain times of the year.

My 5K/10K training was starting and I knew I needed to figure out a way to come to terms with the treadmill. For convenience sake, I tend to use the one in my apartment building, which is in a tiny little room and leaves me feeling all kinds of claustrophobic. When I thought about it, though, I realized that other times on the treadmill, I actually have managed to pull out significant distances and durations without getting bored: the YMCA, hotel gyms, etc. These treadmills had one thing in common: television screens.

Really, it's a sad state of affairs, but it occurred to me that if I had something to focus my attention on, I could basically zone out the physical part of what I was doing and be blissfully entertained. When I started to actually pay attention to my friends who are running ten or eleven or whatever miles on the treadmill, I realized this was their key to survival as well.

To be honest, I kind of felt like an idiot for taking so long to realize this. I mean, is *everyone* doing this? Is this, like, a thing? Some secret understanding that runners just don't talk about? Because, I have to say, in the past I'd use running on the treadmill in the morning as justification for spending my afternoon watching really trashy reality television and now I could do both at the same time?!

So there I was, setting up my tablet on the middle of the console with my show all ready to go. Naturally, I adjusted it so that it was blocking the clock on the treadmill, as I didn't want that distracting me. I had my Garmin watch, which would buzz with each interval and would be enough to keep an eye on the time. I synced the watch and the treadmill and pushed the bright green start button.

And, just like that, before I knew it I was done.

Granted, I was training for a shorter race, so I didn't need any ridiculously long distance, so I'm talking maybe only half an hour worth of work, but in the past that would have been about twenty-five minutes of sheer torture after five minutes of minimal torture; this time it wasn't that bad. In many ways, it reminded me of the very first time I stepped on this treadmill almost exactly four years before. I had some preconceived notions about how I was going to feel during and after, but I was pleasantly surprised to discover I didn't actually hate it after all.

The weeks of training continued, winter transforming yet again into spring and soon I was able to start heading outside again. March brought the annual St. Malachi. This was my fourth year running it, but this year I chose the 2-Mile race as it fit into my training calendar better than the longer 5-Mile race option did. With the staggered start times, I was done before the 5-Mile race even started and I discovered that St. Malachi has a huge finisher's festival at the finish line. All sorts of vendors were set up with both food and drink. I had never been able to take part in the past because by the time I finished running the 5-Mile race, they had all already packed up and left.

Along with outdoor races on the weekends, I also had a new job and a new schedule, both of which left me with a little more creativity to fit runs in during the week.

My previous job had me working four ten-hour work days, although with commutes and lunches built in I was gone twelve hours a day. Now, I worked for a company that not only gave me a more traditional 9-5 schedule, but also fully supported healthy living for the staff. Not only do they offer workout classes during the week at lunchtime, but there is a walking trail out back and a warehouse full of free weights and kettlebells of all sizes and weights. And as if that wasn't enough, there's also a locker room with a full set of showers, which means that people like me—the ones that don't "glow" while working out, but full-on sweat instead—can take a shower and clean up before going back to work for the rest of the afternoon.

BEST. JOB. EVER.

Realizing that I could fit some of my training runs in on my lunch hour was an awe-inspiring moment. The kind of moment that made me sit back and wonder why I hadn't been utilizing my lunch hour for this reason the whole time I'd been here. I mean it was just so *obvious*. Silly Jilly. Granted, because I only get an hour and have to build changing times before and after into that, this plan wouldn't work for very long runs, but with some effort I could get between two and three miles in.

No longer would I have to wake up at some ridiculous hour and run outside in the dark. Also I wouldn't have to spend all day at work with the "I have to run tonight" dread hanging over me. Running on my lunch hour burned off some pent-up energy created by sitting in my cube all day and then I'd come back after lunch ready to push through the second half of the work day.

On the days I wasn't running, I'd take advantage of the Zumba and yoga classes that were offered, creating a built-in, well-rounded running and cross-training program that worked my body and also let me sleep in slightly.

Best of both worlds, amirite?

April brought me the biggest lifestyle change of them all: after seven years of living in downtown Cleveland, nestled on the banks of the Cuyahoga among the machines of industry, I had moved in with my boyfriend and was now living in the neighboring town of Lakewood.

Lakewood is close enough to downtown to still be considered urban, but has a cozy feel that lends itself to feeling equally suburban. (a.k.a. it is also the best of both worlds.) Suddenly I had sidewalks to run on. Lots of them. Sidewalks that seemed to go on for miles and miles and miles.

The best part of this move was that all the city parks were in walking and, well, now running, distance. Before, even when I chose to run at Edgewater or the Metroparks, I'd still have to drive there. Now, I could run to the park, run in the park, then run home from the park. With this new break in my midday and spring allowing for outdoor weekend runs, I no longer had to rely on the treadmill to get my runs in and while I was certainly grateful for an opportunity to get outside and literally pound the pavement, I also knew that this was a short-lived reprieve. Living in Cleveland means that after fall starts, sundown is *wayyy* earlier, and I'll once again have to face that old treadmill. Of course, now that I've moved I won't have to worry about entertaining myself on the one in that small room and can take advantage of the dreadmills at the nearby Y, but either way, now that I have a plan of attack, I feel far less dread when it comes to the dreadmill. We may actually become friends after this.

Well, then again, maybe not. I mean, let's not go all crazy here or anything.

I had started training for the 5K/10K Challenge in early February 2016 and I was so excited to be representing the back of the pack yet again as an Ambassador. I was consistent with my training, getting my long runs in, and following through with weekly cross-training. I was excited to reunite with my running family of fellow Ambassadors and share in our love of this sport. There was the Expo and the VIP dinner and, of course, there was race day. Lining up downtown, the spark and energy that surged through the crowd. I was on a roll, baby.

A couple weeks later, I'd start training for the Akron Half and I was ready to go. I had picked a new training plan, one that focused on speed and would hopefully get me to my PR. Unlike the 2015 Cleveland Half, I was *really* looking forward to training. I'd already written all my runs down in my planner, contacted the local high school about residents using the track during the summer, and started focusing on nutrition more.

Man on mangoberry, I WAS READY TO ROCK AND RUN.

And then a runner's worst nightmare happened.

21

Forward Is Still a Pace

Let me set the scene for you: it's Tuesday, May 10, 2016 at around 6:30 p.m. I get home from a pretty typical day at work and start putting dinner together: baked honey Sriracha chicken thighs with green beans. Ben and I have been living together for a month now. It's a century home full of old wood and lots of character. Not the most up-to-date, but it's gorgeous and it's ours (at least for the next two years, per the terms of our lease).

Ben walks in the door just as I'm putting the chicken in the oven. With the Cleveland Marathon weekend just a few days away (meaning that the 5K and 10K Challenge are just a few days away), I'm being careful with my hydration and nutrition. It's that tricky point of training where it's super easy to give into the concept of carbo loading and instead go way overboard.

Ben heads upstairs and I pull the green beans out of the freezer. When I had first moved in, the freezer was full of frozen vegetables on the point of freezer burn, his roommates apparently not quite as concerned about their daily fruits and vegetable requirements as I am. When they have been over and seen the fridge they are rather impressed with how well stocked I keep it: not just with food, but healthy food.

That's me, the Domestic Goddess.

I put the beans in a pot and head upstairs to take my work clothes off and get my yoga pants on. While upstairs, Ben asks me about the agenda for the weekend. Because of the 5K on Saturday, I have to get to the Expo on Friday night to get my packet and since my sister is coming in from out of town, I'm picking hers up as well. Then there is the VIP Reception for fancy folks, including the Ambassadors. Saturday morning is the 5K. My dad would be bringing my sister Amy into the city Saturday afternoon, then Sunday morning she and I would run the 10K, then immediately head to my parents' house for a family party.

Busy and jam-packed doesn't even begin to describe it.

Realizing the time, I head back downstairs knowing the chicken will be done soon and I still need to turn the stove on for the beans. The hardwood stairs that separate the first and second floor have small rectangular patches on each step that indicate there used to be small carpet squares that ran down the middle but they have been bare for years.

Right near the bottom of the staircase, my left foot slips on the slick hardwood. It happens so fast and I'm so caught off guard, I don't have any time to react before I fall down, right on top of my left ankle.

FUUUUUUUUUUUUUUUUUUUUUUUUUUUCK.

Fuck. Fuck. Fuck.

I don't move for a few seconds, waiting for my body to get grounded so I can assess the situation. I try to give a little twitch of my ankle. Then I burst into tears.

I'm not crying because it hurts—although it does, a lot—I'm crying because I know that because it hurts that means I probably won't be able to walk on it, and if I can't walk on it, then I definitely can't run on it.

FUCK. (Is there any textual equivalent that denotes louder and angrier than all caps? Because that's what I'm trying to convey here. Big, angry, Times Square billboard–sized FUCK.)

Hearing my cries of pain and tears, Ben comes running down the stairs. I'm sitting on the ground floor, tucked next to the couch, my back against the bottom step. He sits a step above me and starts rubbing my shoulders. I am sobbing.

I'm talking full-on ugly crying. Mascara running, blotchy face, there may even have been snot involved. I lean away from my left leg, putting my weight on the right side of my body. I place my hands on the floor, bracing myself, and attempt to stand up.

Fuuuuuuckity fuck fuck fuck.

Unfortunately this isn't foreign territory for me. I have a history of this sort of thing:

- Exhibit A: Falling off the jungle gym in grade school.
- Exhibit B: Tripping in the garage that one summer my dad and I were supposed to go to Mansfield.
- Exhibit C: Falling while unsuccessfully attempting to fulfill a lifelong dream to be a roller derby girl.
- Exhibit D: THE TREADMILL.

This, though, could not have come at a worse time. I mean, seriously. Tuesday night this has to happen? TUESDAY NIGHT before a SATURDAY *AND* SUNDAY RACE.

Flames. Flames on the side of my face.

The oven starts beeping and I ask Ben if he can take the chicken out. He is hesitant to leave me, but I insist. He takes the chicken out and then asks what to do about the green beans on the stove. From my spot on the floor I give instructions as he finishes dinner. With his help, I get up and hobble over to the table and eat my chicken with a side of green beans and salty, salty tears.

As he starts cleaning up, he asks what kind of ice cream I want from a local ice cream shop. I think he's kidding, but he's not. When he leaves to get some scoops, I also ask if he'd be willing to pick up some support stuff for my ankle from a pharmacy.

Because this isn't my first time at the ankle rodeo, I know the drill: RICE. Rest. Ice. Compression. Elevation.

I settle on the couch and prop my foot up on a stack of pillows. Finally, I'm able to put those bags of frozen veggies leftover from the roommates to good use and get comfy with some frozen corn in a towel. For compression, all I have to use is KT tape, but it gets the job done.

Ben returns with ice cream, an ankle compression sleeve, and an air cast.

BEST. BOYFRIEND. EVER.

My sister is now first on my list of people to call because this Sunday was her very first 10K. We were supposed to be running it together and now it looks like she'll be running it alone. I feel awful because this was a big deal for us and we aren't going to be able to partake in it like we planned.

She, of course, completely understands and tells me to take it easy and just rest.

So that is what I did for the next couple days, eventually returning to work near the end of the week. By then I could put some weight on the ankle and was able to walk, albeit with a slight limp. My air cast was pretty noticeable and coworkers kept asking about the ankle, but it was never so bad that I had to resort to the elevator, and I kept taking the stairs as usual.

My running friends told me not to count anything out. I knew the 10K was probably a greater risk, so those 6.2 miles wouldn't be happening, but the 5K was a maybe, even if I just walked it. At the same time, though, I was supposed to start training for Akron in a couple of weeks. Akron was the race I had my eye on—I wanted that PR and it seemed safer, and smarter, to skip both the 5K and 10K and give my ankle time to heal. Therefore, I left work a little early on Friday and headed downtown to the Convention Center for the Expo. I wasn't planning on running, but I still needed to pick up my sister's race packet.

I learned that race weekend as an injured runner is a very different experience. Normally I'd take my time at the expo, but this was very much a get in and get out situation, and I was so grateful to find a parking spot near the entrance. (Although I didn't find a space at first. Some jackass in an SUV squeezed into a spot just as I was backing into it. If not for that whole ankle bullshit I would have gotten out of my car and HELL HATH NO FURY on his ass. It took another loop, crying while driving, before I found a spot that actually ended up being right in front of the main door.)

Saturday morning, instead of running the 5K, I spent the rainy day sleeping in and reading. My dad brought my sister in the afternoon and we hung out at the house, getting tacos for dinner.

I've said it before and I'll say it again: Cleveland weather this time of year can be very unpredictable. So unpredictable that nobody, and I mean nobody, was anticipating snow in mid-May, but in the days and hours leading up to race weekend that was all anyone was talking about. On the one hand, I was so happy I didn't have to run in that shit. On the other hand, all I wanted to do was run and this was probably the only time I ever would be sad about not running in snow and hail and rain and just really horrible weather.

For the second year in a row, Ben offered to play chauffeur for race day (read: Best. Boyfriend. Ever.), waking up far earlier than he needed to on his day off. Originally I was going to wait at the start line with Amy and meet her at the finish line, but the weather was so bad and I was worried about all the walking on my ankle that I asked if she minded if he dropped me off somewhere that would let me see her on the course.

She didn't, but I felt horrible. Not only was I not running the race with her, I was ditching her at the start line. As Ben pulled away and started to head for a spot where he could drop me off, I started crying again.

(No joke, he managed to see me cry more in the span of a week than he had in the entire previous two years we had been together.)

It turns out, along with the pre-race VIP Reception, there was also a post-race VIP Brunch. I'd been invited in 2015, but because of the time frame and because of my pace, I had to miss it and I hadn't planned on going this year, either, because of a family party.

But then, see, my ankle happened and I was going to need somewhere to kill time while Amy was running and I always say my three favorite words are All Day Breakfast . . .

Ben dropped me off as close to Public Square as he could get. Once the race started, they'd turn a couple of corners and run right past me. With any luck I'd be able to spot my sister in the mass of people. Of course, because we got there so early, I still had time to kill and it was wet and cold so it's possible I went to the nearby casino and lost $20, but whatever.

Moving more slowly than usual, I had to give myself plenty of time to get to wherever I needed to go, so when it was getting closer to the start of the race, I made my way from the casino back to Public Square and found a corner. I didn't see Amy, but I did see some of my other racing friends. As I stood there, clapping and cheering, I realized I had never been a spectator at a race before. Wanting to ensure that my fellow runners in the back of the pack were recognized, I stayed on that corner until the police escort drove by.

The hotel where the brunch was being held was a block away so I slowly, very, very slowly, started to walk in that direction. My slow pace had little to do with my ankle and everything to do with the sidewalk being slick. That, combined with my ankle, was a recipe for a disaster.

Because Amy is a faster runner than I am, I had an inkling of how long it would take her to finish. And since I was moving slowly and I needed to give myself ample time to get where I needed to go, I didn't take a long, leisurely brunch. I took the escalator up to the second floor of the Marriott, checked in, and got my plate of fruit, eggs, and bacon. At this point the ballroom was still pretty empty, and most of the other attendees were family members of runners who were waiting until their person was done.

After finishing my brunch, I headed over to the finish line and found a spot along the fence to wait. My sister, like me, has a unique fashion sense when it comes to running and had chosen a bright patterned pair of running tights to wear, so I knew what to look for and spotted Amy soon after she exited the Shoreway ramp. Thanks to my bright green Slytherin hoodie (Harry Potter fan for life, *yo*), she located me at the same time and we waved.

I had my camera waiting and started snapping pictures as she passed by, finishing her first 10K in a little over an hour.

Right near the end there, the hail started to fall in full force and as we found each other and hugged I realized that if I had been able to run today, that's the kind of shitty weather I'd be running in. Cold, solid, drops of water pelting down, stinging me in the face.

Hmm. Maybe this ankle issue wasn't such a bad thing after all.

Here's the thing. Because I'm quite familiar with sprained ankles, I know what they feel like. I also know what they are supposed to look like and this? This looked *horrible.* My entire left foot was bruised, both above and below the anklebone and the whole top of the foot, directly below the toes. I could walk, yes. There was a limp and I was slow, but I could walk, and as the week went on I could put more pressure on it, but still, it looked really, *really* bad.

So the following Monday night, Ben comes home from work and I'm in the kitchen trying to figure out dinner. Five minutes after he walks in the door he mentions that he'd been talking to a coworker about me and she told him that her sister had fallen and had what she thought was a sprained ankle, but later learned it was broken.

Oh, great. That's just want I wanted to hear.

I burst into tears. "Why would you tell me that?"

His face falls, realizing he's just said pretty much the worst possible thing he could have said. "I thought it would help!"

"How is that helping?"

At this point, dinner has been completely forgotten and I'm about five seconds away from getting in the car and driving myself to the hospital for X-rays. Knowing I can be a wee bit impulsive, Ben is patiently trying to talk it through with me. I'm on the couch, ankle propped up, sobbing, and we decide that just for my own sake of sanity we should go.

We live just a few blocks from the Lakewood Hospital. Once a thriving, full-scale facility, due to some local drama, it currently only operates as an Emergency Room while the Cleveland Clinic makes some changes and upgrades to the campus.

Ben dropped me off at the door and I hobbled in while he parked the car. The waiting room was quiet, almost empty, and we only had to wait for maybe ten or fifteen minutes before I was called back.

The nurse went through the list of patient intake questions, including asking my pain level on a scale of ten. I said a one or a two. It was more uncomfortable and annoying than anything else. They asked what brought me in and I said I had fallen the week before and it felt sprained, but looked really bad so I wanted to check just to be sure.

Those were my exact words: "Just to be sure." That said, even with all of my panic half an hour ago, I was feeling pretty confident I'd pay a couple hundred dollars in a co-pay and be sent back with my sprained ankle and maybe a prescription for painkillers. I mean, hello, I'd been walking on the damn thing all week. Even the doctor, when we met, asked if he saw me walking back here on my own. How bad could it be?

Yeah. About that.

In typical emergency room fashion, we were there for about three hours and had maybe twenty minutes of face time with the doctor. But, since we're both librarians, we each came prepared with big books.

About half an hour after I had my X-rays taken, Doctor Andy walked back in.

"So, it's broken. Looking at probably six to eight weeks."

He said this so matter-of-factly that it took my brain a second to process the information. And when it did I, once again, burst into tears.

(The fact that this is all happening about two days before my period no doubt affected the bottomless well of emotions now pouring out through my eyeballs. I'm like fucking Alice in Wonderland over here, drowning in a pool of my own tears.)

Doctor Andy nodded sympathetically. "Did you have something planned?"

"I . . . am . . . a . . . runner," I managed to get out between sobs. "I'm supposed to start training for the Akron Half soon."

His blue eyes widened and his face fell. "Oh, I am so, so sorry," he said, voice soft. "I'm a runner, too. I honestly didn't think it would end up being broken and I was pulling for you. Had I known you were a runner, I would have really been pulling for you."

That runner camaraderie, man. It knows no bounds.

He left for a few minutes and the nurse returned. Seeing my tear-streaked face, she asked if it was because of the pain or because of the situation. (This was the first of many times that people were skeptical when I told them it didn't hurt. Again: *I had walked on it for a week.*)

I said the situation.

She nodded, "Andy talked to you then?"

Yes. Yes he did.

Lakewood Hospital currently didn't have an orthopedic department so all they could do was put me in a splint and send me home with a list of local bone docs to call in the morning, which was Tuesday.

They also sent me home with a prescription for codeine, which, granted, I didn't really need, but I am not one to look a gift horse in the mouth.

By the time we got home it was about 10:30 p.m. and there was no way in hell I was going to make it into work the next day. Ben assured me this was a situation that was an exception to the "Don't call your manager late at night" rule.

Because Ben works late on Wednesdays, we had hoped to get an appointment that morning so he could take me, but the bone doctor prefers patients visit within twenty-four hours of their ER visit. I think they probably mean "within twenty-four hours of the break," in which case I could probably have argued against that, but decided to go along with it. Ben had already left for work so I called my dad, who works downtown Cleveland and has the kind of grown-up executive C-suite–level job that allows for flexibility when your daughter breaks her ankle and needs a ride.

Like Doctor Andy, the bone doctor was rather impressed I'd walked on it for a whole week. Not only that, but that my week of weight-bearing and very little support didn't do any further damage. Because of this, bone doc, a.k.a. Doctor Strimbu, wanted to see what would happen if he gave the ankle full support and no weight-bearing. This meant a full-on cast with a lovely set of crutches to go with it.

Great.

One small gift: I got to pick the color. I chose purple. How sad that this was pretty much the highlight of the experience.

That's not entirely true. I actually got lucky. Very lucky. The non-technical term is a broken ankle, but what I actually had was a closed, non-displaced fracture of the fibula. Well, if I'm being *really* technical, it wasn't my ankle, but my calf bone that I just happened to break down by the ankle. Both Doctor Andy and Doctor Strimbu said this is an injury that comes with a 50 percent chance of surgery and, so far, all signs pointed to being on the good side of 50 percent. Which is saying something seeing as how I spent an entire week *walking on a broken ankle.* Those statistics are, I think, what prompted Doctor Strimbu to take the more extreme recovery option of a cast versus, say, a boot.

But more than that, I'd been running for over four years and this is the first time I'd been injured. All those runs, all those races, miles after miles after miles of training and this was the first time I'd been side-lined. It was another running learning curve, but that's how it goes sometimes. Amirite?

POSTSCRIPT

As of this writing, I still am very much sidelined. This happened in mid-May 2016, and it's now late July 2016. Summer is officially in full swing and the change in weather—a far cry from the snow seen at the Cleveland Marathon weekend—has brought out the runner in everyone. As I sit on the couch, writing, my laptop propped up on my lap, my left foot out in front of me, resting on a stack of pillows, I can look out onto the quiet street in front of the house. Because it's a century home, we don't have central air so we keep the front door open most days when we're home. Runners of all shapes, sizes, and speeds happily pass by. Maybe they are running just for fun, maybe they are a new runner getting their legs out for the first time, or maybe they are training for a fall race. Under different circumstances I would be out there with them, logging the miles. But, well . . .

This is not the end I planned to write. This is not the way the story was supposed to go. But this . . . this is life.

Last year I ran one race per month, which means that by this time last year, I had five races under my hydration belt. Now, I only have that 2-mile St. Malachi. I don't know when I'll walk again, let alone run. Every day is a new challenge that presents new obstacles, although I'm adapting well and discovering necessity really is the mother of invention. That said, from someone who travels not just by walking, but by running as well, this whole forced immobilization thing is a real struggle. From where I sit right now, forward really *is* a pace.

At this point, I may have to completely rewrite my number one rule of running and racing and say that buying race insurance totally trumps reading course maps. You can bet your ass I will be buying it whenever it's offered from here on out. I don't care if it's something as short as a 5K, that insurance will be purchased.

The weeks have turned into months, my leg spending six weeks in a non–weight-bearing cast, then two weeks in a walking cast, and now a boot. I'm at that phase where I come back every couple of weeks for X-rays, a phase that can last for, well, however long it takes to heal, I guess. Eventually physical therapy will be added in but for now, all I can do is take care of my body and wait.

The Akron Half Marathon, now a mere two months away, is so totally not happening.

As it happens, that's the same date as the National Book Festival in Washington, D.C., where Stephen King will be their headliner. Now, because of the injury, I can go. Funny how life works out, eh?

2016 was supposed to be my year. It was the year I was going to really focus, really train, and hit that personal record. But life, as it does, had other plans.

The thing is, I'm not as upset about this now as I was when it first happened. I've finally learned the fine art of patience and the importance of living in the present. I can't change what happened. I don't have a madman in a blue police box popping in and out of my life nor do I have a DeLorean parked out back, waiting to be cranked up to eighty-eight miles per hour.

I can't go back and stop myself from breaking my bone. I can't rewrite history. All I can do is look ahead and keep moving forward, one day at a time.

(If nothing else, because of the broken bone I don't have to be out there running my ass off in ninety degree weather. So, y'know, there are silver linings if I know where to look.)

That said, I was asked to come back as an Ambassador for Cleveland for the third year in a row. Me: the fat, slow, and now injured runner. Those silly race organizers must be out of their minds but at least there is a road to redemption in 2017. Hope really does spring eternal, as *The Shawshank Redemption* reminds us.

I don't know which distances I'll be racing in 2017 because I don't know where I'll be training-wise come January. But I am, surprisingly, optimistic. Cautious, but optimistic all the same. Even if I don't make Cleveland 2017 my fourth half marathon, I have no doubt that with more time, patience, and physical therapy, I'll be running thirteen miles again, hopefully sooner rather than later. There are lots more finish lines in my future and I'll cross them in my own way, at my own pace.

For now, with hundreds of miles behind me and hundreds more still to come, I find myself back at the beginning. Only this time I come armed with the knowledge and experience of a seasoned veteran, not a newbie terrified of stepping on that treadmill for the first time (well, okay, I still maybe get a little gun-shy around the dreadmill, but can you really blame me?). So I step forward into the future the same way I did over four years ago: one foot in front of the other.

Afterword

I'm sitting on the edge of the tub in the home I share with Ben. It's July 2016 and as of about two months ago, I finished the manuscript for my first memoir, *Running with a Police Escort*. The book writing process took an unexpected turn when, instead of finishing up the story championing my crossing the finish line at the Cleveland 10K, I had to deal with a fractured fibula. The injury completely sidelined me and interrupted all training, including the training I had planned on starting soon for the Akron Half-Marathon.

Now, several weeks later, my bone doc had graduated me from a plaster cast to a walking boot and while I wasn't running yet, I was more ambulatory than before. This evening I had attended a concert for my friend Maura's band (the same band quoted at the very beginning of this book). All was going well until partway through the concert when I got up to use the restroom and felt what could only be described a pulled muscle in my groin.

It is important to note that just a few weeks before this, I hauled myself, broken foot and all, to Indianapolis to attend what was to be the final FitBloggin conference. At the 2015 event, I gave an Ignite speech about being a slow runner and at the 2016 event, I led a small group session. (It really was a small group. There were only four of us. And that included myself. Overall attendance of the conference was way down, which most likely contributed to the fact that there has not yet been a conference since).

Anywho. The drive from Cleveland to Indianapolis is about five hours each way and I decided to drive straight through with minimal, if any, stops. I also decided to cut my trip short and return home a day early, also with minimal stops on the way back. For the entire duration of the drives, my left foot, immobilized in the boot, sat firmly planted beneath the steering wheel of my car.

Around the same time as FitBloggin, I had gone on a very big green smoothie kick and every morning I would use my Ninja blender to make myself a smoothie for breakfast using a ridiculous amount of leafy green spinach. (Trust me here. This will become very important information in a minute.)

Right. So. I went to Maura's show and something felt off physically. I stayed, but as the evening progressed my leg started to hurt and it became difficult to walk. When I got home, I told Ben I was going to take a shower and go right to bed.

Which is how I ended up sitting on the edge of our tub, staring at my leg in growing horror. Because when I took the boot off, I discovered that my leg was visibly swollen and discolored. Like purple and blue discolored. Looking like a limb belonging to Voldemort discolored.

Those of you with any medical knowledge may see where this is going, but for those who are lacking in that information, let me help you out. See, injuries often make you susceptible to other medical issues. Like blood clots. Immobilization of limbs exasperates the problem as it reduces circulation. This is why bed-ridden hospital patients are often given compression socks of some variety, to keep the blood flowing even when the patient is unable to move their legs.

Just the weekend before, I had spent ten hours in the car, my leg and foot planted in the same 90-degree angle for the entire duration of the drive. Granted, even on a normal drive when I am not wearing a boot or cast, I still tend to keep my foot planted. The difference is that in those circumstances I also am able to kind of naturally move or fidget my foot and ankle, providing some movement. The boot didn't allow me to do that.

The reason my leg was significantly larger and purple? I had a blood clot. A serious blood clot, which had probably been festering since my road trip to Indianapolis a few days before.

Oh, and the spinach? Leafy green vegetables are full of Vitamin K, a natural coagulant, which means it naturally helps blood clot. In fact, if you're on certain blood thinners and start to have uncontrollable bleeding, you will often be given a shot of Vitamin K to stop it. So at the same time I unknowing have a blood clot brewing, I'm feeding myself significant amounts of Vitamin K, just feeding that blood clot. *Great.*

As I stared at my swollen, purple leg that evening, I was fairly certain I knew what was happening. Of course, I, like most adults of my generation, tend to avoid conflict, and it was late at night, and I was tired and too exhausted to want to deal with it so I just went to bed. I not only went to bed, the next morning I *went to work.*

It was only after getting to the office and struggling to walk to my desk that I realized, hey, maybe I shouldn't be at the office right now and took myself to an urgent care office. The very kind doctor there sent me to the nearest hospital where I walked into the Emergency Room and was seen by Radiology.

Word of advice: if you're ever having an ultrasound done and the technician steps out of the room saying she needs to go get some help, be prepared for very bad news.

The blood clot in my leg ran *literally* the entire length of my left thigh. Literally, the entire length of my thigh. My left leg was severely discolored and the vascular surgeon could only find a teeny bit of a pulse in the very bottom of my foot. I had what was known as Deep Vein Thrombosis, or DVT.

Needless to say, I was taken in for emergency surgery on my leg. I was subsequently taken back into surgery twice more and spent several days hanging out in the Intensive Care Unit. All told, I spent a week in a hospital hooked up to a Heparin drip. All because one evening back in May I tripped on the bottom two steps of our staircase at home.

So, y'know, that was fun.

JUST KIDDING. It was terrible and awful and maybe one day I'll write a book about it. But it's made me stronger, and some good things have happened since then.

In the two years since the publication of *Running with a Police Escort*, I have had the opportunity to attend author events and signings all over the state of Ohio, meeting other runners of all speeds and skills. In that time, two questions come up more frequently than any other: am I still with Ben? And do I have any upcoming races?

As I'm writing this in late 2018, I can tell you that my beloved *Christmas Story* Run is just a few weeks away and I will be running it for the fourth time. This year's theme is Bumpus Hounds, a reference to the rascally dogs who ruin Christmas dinner and force Ralphie and his family to eat Chinese. In the spirit of the theme, the racing organizers have opened up the registration to include dogs as well as humans.

I'll admit, I'm not too crazy about the theme. That said, I love the race and am looking forward to once again hanging out with all the pink bunnies in downtown Cleveland as we make our way to the *Christmas Story* House. I will also admit to you that now, a few years later, I really regret intentionally skipping the race's second year. At the time, I was mostly just focused on how much I disliked the 2014 bling. Today, of course, I'm all, *It would be so cool to be able to say I have run this race every single year.* As in years past, I imagine the upcoming *Christmas Story* Run will be cold and snowy but that's just December in Cleveland, and I wouldn't have it any other way.

Unfortunately, unless Jodie Whitaker shows up with her blue TARDIS and whisks me away across time and space, there's nothing I can do about it.

But, one race I have run every single year since I started is the annual St. Malachi Church Run. I ran it in March 2018 and I can guarantee I'll be running it again in 2019 and beyond.

At last year's race I ran into some women I had met earlier in the year when I had been invited to their book club meeting. They are all local to Cleveland and had chosen *Running with a Police Escort* as one of their monthly picks! 1) How amazing is that? And 2) How cool is it that I got to attend the meeting? (Psst: If your book club is reading my book, I would love to organize an in-person visit or Skype chat! Visit my website at www.jillgrunenwald.com and be sure to reach out so we can set something up.)

After reading *Running with a Police Escort* and talking with me about it, many in the book club had been inspired to adopt the one race a month goal I had set for myself and several members of the group had chosen the *Christmas Story* Run as their December race.

234

Frequently I get emails from readers who share similar inspiration, but this was the first time I'd seen those inspired runners out in the wild, so to speak.

The emails I get from readers are honestly my favorite part about the book writing process because it lets me, as a writer, know that what I said matters. My story matters. But, more than that, the stories of slow runners and walkers and back of the packers *matter*. Over and over again, I receive emails from readers and runners who thank me because my book helped them feel seen as a runner. As a reader, I know how affirming it can be to see yourself on the pages of a book and as a writer it means the world to me to know that I can help other readers and runners feel valued. Readers send me their own stories about running with a police escort and sometimes I even get pictures, the front fender of a police car visible over their shoulder.

When I first wrote *Running with a Police Escort*, I thought it was because I wanted to put my story of the back of the pack into the world. But I was wrong. What I had no way of knowing at the time is that I wrote the book so I could learn all of your stories as well.

Being in the back can often be a lonely endeavor. There's no true pack like there is at the front or the middle, everyone keeping the same pace like a school of fish. Over the years, I've run many races alone for miles and miles. So I know that it can be bleak in the back. It can make you feel forgotten and unimportant. There's nothing worse than crossing the finish line and not receiving your medal, because the race ran out—which happened to me for the very first time in 2017.

The emails I receive from readers like you remind me that I'm not alone, not really. Not even when I'm out there, trudging along by myself like a turtle in a big vat of peanut butter. So thank you for that, all of you. Thank you for consistently reminding me that mile by mile we are all in this together.

Oh, and Ben?
Reader, I married him.

Jill Grunenwald
November 2018

Acknowledgments

Thanks to my editor Ronnie Alvarado and everyone at Skyhorse Publishing. Not to belabor a metaphor but this process was a lot like running a long-distance race and having a dedicated cheering section helped push me through to the end.

Thanks to Alicia Hansen for asking the question, "What would you do if you knew you could not fail?"

Thanks to Andrew Sasak, PA for his compassion and Dr. Victor P. Strimbu for his expertise.

Thanks to the Cleveland Marathon organization and my fellow Ambassadors Andrew Hettinger, Jamie Johnston, Debi Lantzer, Emily Baumgartner, Melissa Bixler, Melissa Carney, Stephani Itibrout, Jessica McCartney, Pam McGowan, Doug Picard, Rachel Frutkin, Joe Fell, Stephanie Lesco, and Christine Cassar. Your love and support means so much and this tortoise is so happy I get to call you amazing hares my friends.

Thanks to Carol Cotten, Christine Radie, Patricia Picard, Sheila Pressler, and Virginia Snyder for always asking "Are you currently writing anything?" long after I left your classrooms.

Thanks to my family, Dave and Sue Grunenwald and Amy and A. J. Burke, who have braved freezing temperatures on more than one occasion to see me cross a finish line.

Finally, and most importantly, thanks to Ben Cox for . . . well, everything, but especially for your sheer awesomeness during the months of #anklegate and all the Mitchell's Ice Cream.

31901064793153